Discover how you can help yourself:

- **Lower cholesterol**
- **Lower blood pressure**
- **Lose weight and keep it off**
- **Save money over diet programs**
- **Protect the health of your heart and**
- **Thereby live longer**

Easy to read charts list percent of calories from fat in over 300 foods. For foods not listed, the "E-Z-2 Read Fat Chart" instantly helps you discover the percent of calories that come from fat. A must for anyone trying to limit fat to less than 30 percent of their calories as recommended by the American Heart Association.

Lose a pound a week like clockwork!

Become an expert on what to eat and not eat to lower your risk of heart disease and cancer.

Joe Mason's program is not based on special foods or supplements—only foods available at your local supermarket. Using this program Joe lowered his cholesterol from 346 to 155. His triglycerides went from 392 to 73. He also lost 35 pounds and kept it off. With the information he passes on to you. "A HEART ATTACK CAN SAVE YOUR LIFE."

This book is available at special quantity discounts for bulk purchases for sales promotions, premiums, fund raising, or educational use.

For details, write or telephone
Special Markets
Readers Choice
2141 Shaw Ave., Suite 1212
Clovis, CA. 93611-8916
(209) 298-8062

Please write to the author with suggestions or comments to the above address. The author is especially interested in low-fat, healthy recipes for a future book.

800 SERVICE

For fast service, order this book by calling America West Books at 1-800-497-4909. We are sorry but no discounts or special offers are available through the 800 number. See back of the book for special offers by mail.

A Heart Attack

Can

Save Your Life!

The complete guide on how to lose weight and reduce your risk of heart attack and cancer without dieting.

by Joseph W. Mason

Although the author and publisher have exhaustively researched all sources to ensure the accuracy and completeness of the information contained in this book, we assume no responsibility for errors, inaccuracies, omissions, or any inconsistency herein. Any slights of people or organizations are unintentional. Readers should use their own judgment or consult their personal physicians for specific applications to their individual problems.

Library of Congress Catalog Card Number:
95-67488

Publisher's Cataloging in Publication Data
Mason, Joseph W.
A Heart Attack Can Save Your Life: The complete guide on how to lose weight and reduce your risk of heart attack and cancer without dieting / by Joseph W. Mason
Bibliography: p.
Includes index
1. Diet, low fat
2. Health
3. Nutrition
4. Heart Disease
5. Cholesterol
RM222.   1996   613.2   LC95-67488
ISBN 0-9646109-4-9 $15.95 Softcover

TABLE OF CONTENTS

TABLE OF CONTENTS

INTRODUCTION:

Who Is This Book For?

If you are overweight, have high cholesterol, or want to reduce your risk of heart attack and cancer this book is for you. It will provide you with know-how to make lifestyle changes that will decrease your risk of heart disease and some cancers.

After my heart attack, I was surprised to find out during my rehabilitation how little I knew about the heart, cholesterol, calories, nutrition, and exercise. As I increased my knowledge through study and research, it seemed almost too easy to lower my weight and my cholesterol.

The key is knowledge. You can't perform any meaningful job or do any worthwhile task without it. You can't drive a car, bake a cake, or fly an airplane without being knowledgeable in that particular area. So, how can people protect their health if they have little or no knowledge about nutrition? And, by the way, food manufacturers don't help. When they slap "80 percent fat free" across a food label of a product that gets 76 percent of its calories from fat, it's no wonder we're confused. It's time for you to become informed. Your health depends on it.

The knowledge I gained is shared in this book. I describe how to lose weight easily and safely and how to lower your cholesterol. Exercise information is discussed in detail.

1

A HEART ATTACK CAN SAVE YOUR LIFE

How can I say it is easy? Well, a few years ago a friend taught me how to do a tune up on my car. It was easy once I had the know-how. It's the same with being overweight. I talked to many people who say they are trying to lose weight and are on some diet or weight loss program. But when I ask them a few simple questions, they know almost nothing about nutrition. I don't think you can lose weight and keep it off without knowledge concerning nutrition.

The same is true about cholesterol. Not many people know their cholesterol level. And for those who do, often the extent of their knowledge is that eggs are bad for them. This falls far short of what they should know to be heart attack safe.

This book is for the millions of men and women struggling against weight and high cholesterol levels who are interested in improving their health. It accomplishes this very simply by providing information to educate and make you knowledgeable. Throughout the book there are easy to answer questions. They're easy because the answers are found in *italics* in the text. Writing down the answer is a good way to retain this information, which is the objective in learning. Now is the time for you to discover how to safely improve your health.

I suggest that you read the whole book before you start applying any of it to your daily living. Then go back to reread the parts that pertain to you. This is not a diet book. In fact, if you follow the guidelines you will get to eat more. You may not need to lose weight, but you may be interested in lowering your cholesterol. Or perhaps you are wondering how nutrition and exercise can help to prevent heart disease. In short, weight, cholesterol, nutrition, and exercise go hand in hand to affect your health and longevity. Isn't it time you learned about your health? Don't you want to live longer?

This book is also for doctors, educators, and counselors— any professionals who want to pass on to their patients, students, or clients information in easily understood terms that will increase their knowledge.

This book will save you money too. You won't need to join an exercise club, buy special foods, or join some weight loss program. In fact, as you'll learn, some of these can be dangerous to your health. In this book you will discover how to lose weight safely.

INTRODUCTION

In a nutshell, I have tried to include in one book all the information you will need to start a heart maintenance program for a healthier life. Included are special charts and food listings that will make it easier for you to understand nutritional information.

Are you tired of seeing the word knowledge? I've used this word seven times so far. Why? Because being knowledgeable about a subject is what allows us to succeed. There is a direct relationship between how much you know about a subject and how successful you are in accomplishing an endeavor. In summary, the three most important elements of a heart maintenance program are knowledge, knowledge, and knowledge.

Before you go on you may find it helpful to skim through the glossary for unfamiliar terms.

I hope you find the reading interesting and the material helpful. I wish you a long and pleasurable life.

WHEN YOU
UNDERSTAND
YOU CAN SUCCEED

THE ESSENCE OF
KNOWLEDGE IS,
HAVING IT, TO USE IT—
Confucius

CHAPTER 1

Your Good Health Depends On What You Know

In 1985, at the ripe old age of 41, a massive heart attack almost ended my life. Six years later, after my annual exercise test, my cardiologist said: "In terms of fitness, you are in the top five percent of males your age who haven't had a heart attack."

How did I turn my health and life around? How did I lower my weight by 35 pounds, from 175 to 140? How did I lower my cholesterol from 346 to 155? I did it by learning what I could do to protect my heart. A heart attack truly did save my life.

It's no wonder I had a heart attack, I knew nothing of heart maintenance. I fit Will Rogers statement, "We are all ignorant—only on different subjects." I had tried for 15 years to lose ten pounds. After becoming "un-ignorant," I lost 35 pounds and I was eating more.

Let's test your knowledge to see what you know and what more you need and can learn.

What is your weight? _____
What is your ideal weight? _____ (see appendix)
Are you overweight? _____ If, yes, by how much? ___
What is your cholesterol level? _____
What is your High Density Lipoprotein level? _____
What is your Low Density Lipoprotein level? _____
What is your blood pressure? _____
What is your resting pulse? _____
What does an aerobic exercise mean? _____

Do you know what exercises build a strong heart?

Do you know how to lose one pound a week while you
actually eat more? _____
Do you understand all the information on a food label?
_____
What does 97 % fat free mean? _____
What is your target heart rate? _____

 After following the guidelines in this book you will be able
to answer these questions and the information will help you
control your weight and cholesterol.
 Let's discuss cholesterol next, since it appears to be the
most important topic when we talk about heart disease.

WHY NOT CULTIVATE
HEALTH
INSTEAD OF
TREATING DISEASE ?

CHAPTER 2

The Predictor Of Heart Disease

Most people don't know their cholesterol level. More than half of all Americans have blood cholesterol levels high enough to be at risk for heart disease, but less than 10 percent of the population even knows their cholesterol levels. At the time of my heart attack, in 1985, I wasn't even familiar with the word cholesterol. Of course, it wasn't the household word it is today.

The link between high cholesterol levels and heart disease is indisputable. All over the world in countries where the people have a low blood cholesterol level, they also have a low incidence of coronary artery disease. Almost no one with a long-term cholesterol level below 160 mg/dl develops heart disease. (mg/dl - The weight of cholesterol, in milligrams, in a deciliter of blood. A deciliter is about one-tenth of a quart.) There is also growing evidence that lowering one's cholesterol below 160 mg/dl will actually *reduce the cholesterol already built up in the arteries.* In order to combat this enemy you need to know what cholesterol is and how it gets in your blood.

Cholesterol is a soft, waxy substance that is essential to our well-being. It is used for the manufacture of hormones, bile acid, and vitamin D.

Cholesterol is found in all animals. Any food that comes from an animal contains cholesterol: meat, fish, eggs, milk, and dairy products. Foods that come from plants do not contain cholesterol: fruits, vegetables, grains (wheat, oats, rice).

The liver manufactures cholesterol in sufficient quantity for normal body functions, even when we consume no cholesterol at all. Beside cholesterol in your food, the saturated fat we eat encourages the liver to produce more cholesterol.

In rare cases the liver makes more cholesterol than it should. You may have no symptoms though this extra cholesterol may slowly clog your arteries. In fact, the first indication of something being wrong could be a fatal heart attack. A six year old girl from Texas is one such notable case. She had a cholesterol level over 1,000 mg/dl and had a heart attack. She ended up needing a heart and liver transplant. This is one good reason to have a blood cholesterol test, just to make sure your liver is functioning normally.

Cholesterol travels in your blood stream in packages called LIPOPROTEINS. The cholesterol and fat, known as lipids, do not mix well with blood. In order for these lipids to travel through the blood stream, your liver wraps the lipids in proteins forming lipoproteins. In very simple terms, VERY LOW-DENSITY LIPOPROTEINS (VLDL) carry fat and cholesterol out of the *liver* and to all parts of the *body*. The VLDL distribute the fat they carry throughout the body. What is left is called a *LOW DENSITY LIPOPROTEIN* (LDL). The LDL is rich in *CHOLESTEROL*. The LDL then travel back to the liver where they are either recycled into new VLDL or broken down and excreted. This is the way it works in a person with ideal blood cholesterol levels.

If you eat too much CHOLESTEROL and SATURATED FAT your liver makes extra VLDLs. The original process continues with the VLDLs distributing the fat and becoming LDL. Now comes the problem. Your liver cannot process these extra LDLs, and these cholesterol rich LDLs end up stuck along blood vessel walls. This clogging of the arteries is known as *atherosclerosis*. When an artery of our heart is blocked, it can lead to a *heart attack*, and when an artery to our brain is blocked, it can lead to a stroke.

There is good news though! Studies have concluded that by reducing your blood cholesterol level *you may reverse atherosclerosis.* In other words, the deposits that collected inside your arteries may actually be reduced and taken away.

It would be wise then to keep your VLDL and LDL at a low value. How low? *VLDL should be less than* 30 mg/dl and *LDL should be less than* 130 mg/dl. And your *total cholesterol should be less than* 200 mg/dl.

Another type of cholesterol is called *HIGH-DENSITY LIPOPROTEIN (HDL).* Known as the "good" cholesterol, HDL is capable of bringing the stuck LDL cholesterol back to the liver, but only if your LDL level is not excessive. HDL should be over 35 mg/dl.

So how do you keep the total cholesterol, VLDL and LDL low, and the HDL high? The bad cholesterol can be lowered by reducing the saturated fat and cholesterol in your diet. The good cholesterol can be raised by maintaining your ideal weight and becoming physically active.

Don't think that cholesterol tests are expensive or you need a doctor to order the blood test. Many hospitals offer low cost cholesterol tests. A hospital in my area offers cholesterol tests once a month for five dollars.

Knowing your cholesterol level is the first step in preventing heart disease.

Questions you now can answer:
1. What is cholesterol? _____
   _____
2. Cholesterol travels in your blood stream in packages called? _____
3. Very low-density lipoproteins (VLDL) carry fat and cholesterol out of the _____ and to all parts of the _____.
4. After VLDL distribute the fat they carry they are called _____.
5. LDL are rich in _____.
6. If you eat too much _____ and _____ _____ the liver makes extra VLDL.
7. When too many LDL get stuck along artery walls it's called _____.
8. A blocked artery can cause a _____ _____ or a stroke.

9. By reducing your cholesterol level you may reverse _____.
10. Ideal cholesterol levels are:
   Total cholesterol less than _____.
   LDL less than _____.
   VLDL less than _____.
   HDL more than _____.

```
THE BEST WEALTH
IS
HEALTH
```

CHAPTER 3

Discover How To Help Control Your Cholesterol Level

If cholesterol is a predictor of heart disease and what we eat is a predictor of cholesterol level, it would be prudent to have some knowledge about the food we eat.

Most people know that eggs are high in cholesterol, but that's the extent of their knowledge.

The American Heart Association recommends limiting yourself to 100 milligrams (mg) of cholesterol per 1,000 calories a day with a maximum of 300 mg. cholesterol.

DAILY CALORIES	MAXIMUM CHOLESTEROL
1,000	100 mg
2,000	200 mg
3,000	300 mg

Most people will consume between 1,200 and 2,500 calories per day.

The dietitian on the staff at my cardiac rehabilitation program recommended limiting cholesterol intake to 200 mg. per day for anyone with my history of heart disease or someone with a high blood cholesterol level. To make an effort to control your cholesterol intake, you first need to know your blood cholesterol level.

This is why I'm against the numerous diets that tend to put everyone in the same category. It's important to have knowledge about nutrition, and make the choices that allow you to obtain an ideal cholesterol level and weight that fit you personally and not just any diet or a general one will fit your particular needs.

Cholesterol in the food you eat is not the only thing that raises your blood cholesterol readings. *Saturated fat* raises blood cholesterol more than anything else we eat, even cholesterol. Saturated fat stimulates the liver to make cholesterol.

So now you see, it's important to know about cholesterol and also about fat in food if we expect to have an ideal blood cholesterol level. If you take just 15 minutes a day for 30 days, you can become an expert on what to eat and not to eat in order to lower your risk of heart disease.

Questions you now can answer:
1. The American Heart Association recommends you limit yourself to _____ milligrams of cholesterol per 1,000 calories a day with a maximum of _____ mg. cholesterol.
2. _____ _____ raises blood cholesterol more than anything else we eat.

**WHATSOEVER WAS THE FATHER
OF DISEASE,
AN ILL DIET
WAS THE MOTHER**

CHAPTER 4

Change Your Habits In Only 15 Minutes A Day

My dietitian showed me an easy way to keep track of what I eat. You can use this system in different ways. You can monitor calories, cholesterol, or fat. It takes only 15 minutes each day, and it will make you very knowledgeable. After one to three months you shouldn't need to do it any longer, because you will have established better eating habits. I used it and lost one pound a week like clockwork while I literally ate more.

At the back of this book is a log to write down what you eat each day. There is also a sample list for breakfast, lunch, supper, and dessert. You should add the things you eat to these lists. These lists will allow you to expedite looking up what you eat each day. At the end of the day, add up whatever you are keeping track of. It's obvious that thin people won't need to keep track of calories but they may want to lower their cholesterol.

My wife wanted to lose 15 pounds. Her cholesterol level was good, but she had little knowledge about food. I had her write down everything she ate for one week and give me the list. She was eating a couple of items, almost daily, that derived 50 to 70 percent of their calories from fat. I told her this was going to be easy to change, and she would lose a half to one pound a week. I advised her to only eat these high fat foods on Friday. Everyone should have a party day. On the other days, I substituted foods she liked but ones that were much lower in fat. And because they were lower in fat, she could eat more. She lost her 15 pounds gradually and couldn't believe that she had been trying to do this for nine years, in fact, ever since our twins were born. She could not do it before, because she was not knowledgeable about food.

You may not need or want to keep track of everything. It may be enough for you just to become aware of those few items that are high fat items and that keep you from losing weight or lowering your cholesterol. Everyone is different. Whether you track calories, grams of fat, or cholesterol, or just want to increase your knowledge about a food, the information is here.

> EAT TO LIVE
> NOT
> LIVE TO EAT

CHAPTER 5

It's Easy To Lose Weight If You Like To Eat

In fact, the more things you like to eat, the easier it is to lose weight. The secret is knowing what percent of calories come from fat in the foods you eat. Luckily, I like just about everything. So once I knew what was high in fat, it was easy to substitute something else. Because what I substituted was low in fat, I could eat more.

Here is a simple example. Let's say your stomach is the size of two cups. If you put two cups of anything in your stomach, it will be full. Imagine putting two cups of whole milk in your stomach versus two cups of non-fat milk. In both instances your stomach is full, but take a look at these figures.

2 Cups	CHOLESTEROL (MG)	FAT grams	PERCENT CALORIES FROM FAT	TOTAL CALORIES
Whole Milk	66	16.4	49	300
Non-Fat Milk	8	.8	5	172
Savings by using Non-Fat milk	58	15.6		128
Savings in one Year	21,170	5,694		46,720

Each time your stomach had the same volume of food placed in it, but the calories were almost cut in half by using non-fat milk (172 calories for non-fat milk and 300 calories for whole milk). In addition, the grams of fat were twenty times more for whole milk than non-fat milk (16.4 grams of fat in whole milk compared to .8 grams of fat in non-fat milk). Whole milk gets 49 percent of its calories from fat, while non-fat milk gets only five percent of its calories from fat.

Later in the book you will learn how easy it is to determine the percent of fat calories. Whole milk is what's known as calorie dense and fat dense compared to non-fat milk. With the help of this book you will learn to spot these fat dense foods.

If you drink two cups of milk a day, you will save 128 calories by using non-fat milk (300 calories for whole milk minus 172 calories for non-fat milk equals 128 less each day). This 128 calories times one year (365 days) equals 46,720 calories less each year. As you will learn later in the book, one pound of body fat is equal to about 3,500 calories. So, if you divide the 46,720 calories you save in a year by 3,500 it equals 13 pounds. If you switched from whole milk to non-fat milk you would lose about 13 pounds in a year. If it isn't your goal to lose weight, then you will have 128 calories each day for something else to eat.

Of course you will also save 58 mg. of cholesterol (66 mg. in whole milk and only 8 mg. in non-fat). That's 21,170 mg. cholesterol less in one year (58 X 365). Plus the fact that whole milk has 20 times more fat and saturated fat raises blood cholesterol more than anything.

I know you don't fill your stomach with two cups of milk or two cups of any one item. I know we all fill up with a variety of foods. But if that variety is high in fat, the results are the same. You cannot fill your stomach with foods that get 40 percent or more of their calories from fat and expect to lose weight or lower your cholesterol. You need to know what percent of your calories come from fat. That's made easy with a chart in this book. I know it's easy because my ten year old daughter can read the chart.

Before I go on, it's worth talking about switching to non-fat milk. I didn't think I'd ever switch. The one time I did try non-fat milk, years ago, it tasted like water. Now whole milk tastes like chalk to me. We can modify our taste buds. If you drink whole milk, mix it 50/50 with two percent milk (which is two percent fat by weight but actually gets about 35 percent of its calories from fat). After awhile decrease the amount of whole milk, and before long it will all be two percent milk. Gradually do the same with non-fat milk. I'll bet your taste buds won't know the difference. During the summer I like my milk over ice cubes but that's my personal choice.

I am an advocate of non-fat milk for a couple of reasons. For some people this is all they may need to do to lose 13 pounds a year. As most people know, milk is a very good source of calcium and protein. What many people don't know is that milk is not only a good source of protein, but it is a "high-quality protein," which means it can be combined with other foods that do not contain complete protein to maximize their benefit. I'll discuss this in the chapter about protein.

Of course, I won't discuss each food item you may eat, but I will provide you with the information to make healthy choices. With the knowledge to make wise choices, it will become easy to lose weight if you like to eat.

YOU CAN DO ANYTHING

YOU WANT

IF YOU STICK TO IT

LONG ENOUGH

CHAPTER 6

You Can't Live Without 'EM

Calories are the good guys; without them we'd die. Our body uses calories for fuel just like a car uses gas. These calories make our muscles work and provide the energy for the brain to think. The body burns calories twenty-four hours a day, even while we sleep.

A technical definition for *calories* has to do with giving off heat and can be found in the glossary. For now, it's enough for us to know that a calorie is a unit of energy and is the fuel our body burns. Calories combine with oxygen and give off heat; hence, the term "burning off calories."

Another term you should be familiar with is *nutrient*. A nutrient is a substance obtained from food and used in the body to promote growth, maintenance, and/or repair. The *essential nutrients are* those the body cannot make for itself in sufficient quantities but which it has to obtain from food. The six classes of nutrients are *water, minerals, vitamins, protein, fat, and carbohydrates.*

Did you know your body parts are continuously being replaced by a process which uses nutrients? It's true! You don't have the same skin you had just a few years ago. All the cells are different. These cells were replaced over the years. Even the oldest red blood cell in your body is only six months old. Your body is a perpetual cell maker, and these cells make up all your body parts.

The material to make these new cells has come from your food. As the old saying goes, "you are what you eat." When the foods you eat do not contain the required nutrients, you fail to function as well as you should. In some instances, you may ruin your health, or even die.

Only three nutrients supply calories (energy): *fat, protein, and carbohydrates*. Everyone needs some of each of these nutrients to stay healthy. Almost all foods contain mixtures of all three energy nutrients. Many foods are high in one nutrient and contain just a small amount of the other two. Fruits and vegetables are high in carbohydrates with a small amount of protein and a trace of fat. Exceptions to this are avocados and coconut, both high in fat.

Fat, protein, and carbohydrates supply different amounts of calories for their weight.

> 1 Gram of Fat-------------------equals 9 calories
> 1 Ounce of Fat------------------equals 252 calories
> 1 Pound of Fat------------------equals 4,032 calories
> 1 Gram of Carbohydrate-------equals 4 calories
> 1 Ounce of Carbohydrate------equals 112 calories
> 1 Pound of Carbohydrate------equals 1,792 calories
> 1 Gram of Protein -------------equals 4 calories
> The rest of Protein is the same as Carbohydrates.

During metabolism they are broken down at different rates. Metabolism is the body process by which nutrients are broken down to yield energy.

> *Carbohydrate, simple* (sugar)
>> takes 15 to 45 minutes.
>>> Fruits.
>
> *Carbohydrate, complex* (starch)
>> takes 1 to 2 hours.
>>> corn, potato, grain, peas, rice.
>
> *Protein*
>> takes 3 to 4 hours.
>>> meat, milk, eggs.
>
> *Fat*
>> takes 6 to 8 hours to burn up.
>>> nuts, olives, butter, veg. oil.

The above information is very important, and I have included it in Appendix 12 so you can tear it out and post it in a handy place.

The rate or speed with which a nutrient begins to provide energy is critical. A wise selection of the foods you eat depends on this knowledge. A diabetic knows what food gets into the blood the fastest: simple carbohydrates.

If you are hungry, eating something high in fat won't turn off the hunger because fat takes too long to get absorbed into your system. Did you ever eat something, like peanuts or potato chips, that you thought should stop those hunger pangs, only to remain hungry? What you needed to eat was some carbohydrates first.

Here's an example. At noon you have a small lunch of about 300 calories. At two in the afternoon you are hungry. What do you do? Do you starve yourself until supper time at five p.m.? Do you eat some peanuts? Or do you eat an apple? Well, no food program should starve you. NONE! Do not go on a diet that starves you. As you may have learned already, the peanuts are high in fat, and from the preceding information the fat will not kick in as a fuel for some time. You are hungry now, so you need the apple or some other carbohydrate.

Remember the saying about eating a Chinese dinner and how you're hungry again an hour later? It's kind of like all those diets where all you get is a salad, and you're hungry again in an hour. You are just getting carbohydrates, and they are all burned up after a short time. Compare stuffing yourself on a Chinese dinner to stuffing yourself on Thanksgiving dinner. Each time your stomach was filled to the limit, but unlike the Chinese dinner, the Thanksgiving dinner had a lot of fat in it. It takes a long time for all that fat to get broken down and burned up.

You have to learn how to fill your stomach with the correct amounts of carbohydrates, protein, and fat. You can fill your stomach so you won't be hungry in one or two hours, but you won't feel stuffed two hours after you eat either. You need the *right combination* of carbohydrates, protein, and fats. In order to get the right amount of each item, you need to be knowledgeable about what you eat. On some diets people are hungry all the time. This should not happen if you learn to eat the correct items. In fact, when I started to eat correctly, I could not believe I had so much to eat.

In some countries the people do not have the variety of food we have, and they end up not getting one or more of the important vitamins or minerals. This deficiency then leads to illness and disease. In other countries food is not plentiful, and this leads to malnutrition. In the United States we are very fortunate when it comes to food. We have a great variety of food, and most foods are plentiful. This could also be our downfall. We, as adults, pick what we eat like children would if you turned them loose in the supermarket. They would probably start with the candy and ice cream. We'd start with the fat. Oh, we aren't stupid. We know fruit and vegetables are good for us, but we just aren't as knowledgeable as we should be. At least I fell into that category. If we all increase our knowledge as consumers, we will be healthier, wiser shoppers as well as eaters.

We need to make sure we get a variety of food. In the chapter on "Diet," I will discuss variety. We also want to make sure we don't feel starved. We want to learn to eat wisely so we can be as healthy as possible and live as long as possible. We want to keep our arteries clear and thus help avoid heart problems.

You Can't Live Without 'EM

Questions you now can answer:
1. A calorie is _____
   _____
2. A _____ is used in the body to promote growth, maintenance, and repair.
3. The six classes of nutrients are _____,
   _____, _____,
   _____, _____
   _____.
4. What three nutrients supply calories? _____,
   _____, _____.
5. The body process by which nutrients are broken down to yield energy is called _____.
6. 1 ounce of fat equals _____ calories.
   1 ounce of protein equals _____ calories.
   1 ounce of carbohydrates equals _____ calories.
7. Simple carbohydrates take _____ minutes to start providing energy.
8. Complex carbohydrates take _____ to burn up.
9. Protein takes _____ hours to burn.
10. Fat takes _____ hours to burn up.

KNOWLEDGE IS

THE KEY

TO SUCCESS

CHAPTER 7

The Proven Healthy Food

The first body fuel I will discuss is carbohydrates. They are one of the three nutrients that supply calories (energy) to the body. Carbohydrates provide four calories per gram and are divided into either simple or complex depending on how their atoms are composed. They are essential for normal body function. *Carbohydrates* are absorbed into the bloodstream and go to work as fuel faster than protein or fat.

The simple carbohydrates are *sugars*, and the complex carbohydrates are *starches*. All starchy foods are plant foods, with seeds being the richest. The starches that supply most of the world's food energy are the grains. There are a few different staple grains. In the United States, Canada, and Europe, the staple grain is *wheat*. In the Orient, the staple grain is *rice*. In Mexico and South America, the staple grain is *corn*. Some other important grains are barley, rye, millet, and *oats*. These grains are made into flour, meal, or bread.

You only have to read any cereal box to see any of the first group of starches. In America, we have a wide variety of grains in our cereals and breads.

Another very important source of starch is the *bean* and *pea family*. These are important because they are also high in *protein*. If you are cutting back on meat because your cholesterol is high, you will also be cutting back on protein. A good way to get the protein back is with beans and peas. Here's where that knowledge comes into play. I make two delicious soups, pea and bean. In each I get only about one ounce of ham in a serving, so I cut way back on my cholesterol and fat intake, but I don't miss out on my protein.

A third source of starch is the tubers, such as the potato, yam and cassava. These are a major source of starch in some countries.

As I said previously, the simple carbohydrates are the sugars. Besides common white sugar, many of the fruits and vegetables are made up of these sugars. Don't avoid these, because they do contain other nutrients. White sugar, however, has been termed an empty calorie. It provides calories but no other nutrients. (Again that does not mean to avoid sugar, just be knowledgeable about its roles.)

I use a teaspoon of sugar every morning in my coffee. How many calories in a teaspoon of sugar anyway? Fifteen! I don't think that will kill me. I did give up or cut back on a lot of other sweet items when I learned that a high blood triglyceride level was linked to excessive sugar. (Triglycerides are a fat-like substance found in the blood that may be a possible indicator of heart disease.) I would gladly give up the teaspoon in my coffee if my triglyceride level was still high. My triglycerides went from 392 at the time of my heart attack to 73, four years later. This is why I keep saying the first step is to get your blood tested and then make dietary changes based on the blood test results and your weight. Your goal should be to attain an ideal weight and ideal blood test while you are eating foods you like and enjoy.

Dietary intake patterns in the United States have shifted markedly in this century. Carbohydrates were clearly the dominant source of energy in the past but, at the present time, carbohydrates and fats make nearly equal contributions to the energy content of the national diet.

It is recommended that we get *approximately 58 percent of our calories from carbohydrates*, with 10 percent coming from simple carbohydrates and 48 percent coming from complex carbohydrates.

No discussion of carbohydrates would be complete without mentioning that carbohydrates are the main source for glucose. *Glucose* is a simple sugar also known as *blood sugar*. What's important about this fact is that your brain and nervous system require glucose for their *energy*. This fact becomes critical as you learn about protein, fat, and weight control.

Questions you now can answer:
1. _____ go to work to fuel our body faster than protein or fat.
2. Simple carbohydrates are known as _____.
3. Complex carbohydrates are known as _____.
4. A few grains that are complex carbohydrates are: _____, _____, _____, and _____.
5. An important source for complex carbohydrates is _____ and _____, because these are high in _____.
6. ____ percent of our calories should come from _____.
7. Carbohydrates are the main source for _____ also known as _____ _____.
8. Your brain and nervous system require _____ for their _____.

CARBOHYDRATES -   1 Gram = 4 calories;
                    1 ounce = 112 calories.
          SIMPLE - 15 minutes or faster to provide
              energy; Fruits (sugars)
          COMPLEX - Burns in 1 to 2 hours; Pasta,
              Grains (wheat, oats), (Starches)

FLOW CHART FOR CARBOHYDRATES AS THEY ENTER OUR BODY

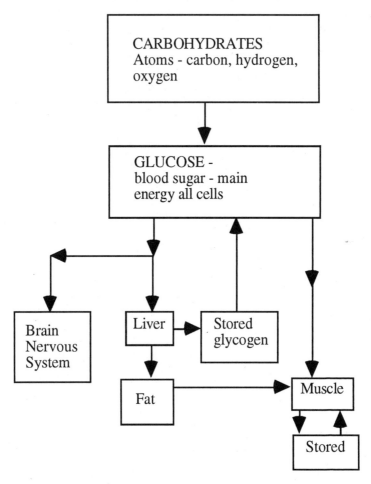

Blood glucose normally 70 - 120 mg.; Below 65 mg. you feel hungry. You eat. Blood glucose rises. Pancreas releases insulin so cells can use glucose. Liver and muscles store glucose in long chains of GLYCOGEN (turn back to glucose as needed), liver also converts glucose to fat. Fat can not convert back to glucose. Stored glycogen is limited, stored fat is not. Fat can not supply the brain and nervous system with energy.

CHAPTER 8

What's Building Your Cells Is Important

Protein is one of the three nutrients that supplies calories to the body. Protein provides four calories per gram, which is less than half the calories of fat. It is also an essential nutrient that becomes a component of many parts of the body, including muscle, bone, skin, and blood. If you are looking for a definition of protein, a chemist might say it's a chemical compound made up of the following atoms: carbon, hydrogen, oxygen, and nitrogen. We are not so interested in what atoms make up protein but what characteristics or qualities protein has once we eat it. In other words what does protein do in our body?

Protein takes about 3 to 4 hours, a longer time than carbohydrates, to get into the blood supply and start providing energy. Meat, milk, and eggs are good sources of protein. Just remember the protein is in the egg white, and the cholesterol is in the yolk. BUT, the protein's first role is not as an energy source. What is protein's main role?

It might help to divide protein into food protein and body protein. We eat food protein so our body can make body protein; however, this is not a direct transfer.

Food protein contains *amino acids*. Amino acids are a compound of the atoms, mentioned earlier, combined in different ways. There are twenty-two different amino acids. Each food protein varies in the amount of amino acids it contains.

The body breaks down these amino acids and combines them in a different order to make body protein. Some chains of amino acids link up with other chains to form giant proteins. There are thousands of different kinds of protein in the body. *All body cells contain protein.* As I said earlier, these cells are constantly being repaired and replaced. This makes amino acids from food protein critical to good health. So, *food protein's main role is to eventually become body protein.*

Some foods are called *quality protein* because they contain the right amino acids in the correct amounts for the body to turn into body protein. Other protein rich foods that do not fit this category can be combined to make quality protein. The table that follows will help you do this. This table also appears in Appendix 13. Tear it out and post it somewhere handy.

For Quality Protein * from vegetable sources, use any food from column 1 in combination with a food from column 2.

	Column1	**Column2**
LEGUMES	BEANS: Adsuki, Black, Cranberry, Fava, Kidney, Limas, Pinto, Marrow, Mung, Navy, Pea, Soy, (Tofu) (Sprouts)	Low-fat dairy products
	PEAS: Black-eyed, Chick Cow, Field, Split LENTILS	Grains Nuts & Seeds
GRAINS	WHOLE GRAINS: Barley; Corn (cornbread) (grits) Oats; Rice; Rye, Wheat (Bulgur, Wheat Germ) Sprouts	Low-fat dairy products Legumes
NUTS & SEEDS	NUTS; Almonds, Beechnuts, Brazil nuts, Cashews, Filberts, Pecans, Pine nuts (Pignolia), Walnuts SEEDS: Pumpkin, Sunflower	Low-fat dairy products Legumes

* *Low-fat dairy products* (milk, yogurt, cheese, eggs, cottage cheese), in addition to being used as a supplement to the above, may be used alone as "quality protein."

Up to now protein sounds great. After all, the protein we eat is replacing the protein we are losing. All we have to remember is some foods need to be combined to get their full benefit. Then why not go on a high protein diet? This is evidently what took place during the 1970's when some deaths were linked to high protein diets. Scientists who studied the deaths found that the dieters had died of irregular heart rhythms and cardiac arrest.

When you take in more protein than you need for cell repair and replacement, you have an excess of amino acids. These amino acids are broken down by the liver to provide energy or to make fat, in a process called "deamination." When the liver has too much to process it ends up releasing large amounts of the toxic compound "urea" into the blood. The urea is processed by the kidneys and excreted in the urine.

This can be very stressful on the *liver* and *kidneys* as they work overtime to rid the body of the toxic urea. Also, in order to dilute the urea you will need to consume large amounts of water and your body may even take water from its own tissue. It is this water taken from the tissue that is the weight loss people experience when they go on a high protein diet. *Two cups of water weighs about one pound.* It is only temporary weight loss because the tissue wants that water back. It only gave up the water to keep the toxic level under control.

There are times when you might want to consume a little more than the Recommended Dietary Allowance (RDA) for protein. If you remember, that, protein is used for repair and replacement of cells, it is easy to understand, if you are sick or have an operation, your doctor may want you to receive a little higher amount of protein. Also, if you are a bodybuilder you are interested in increasing the size of your muscles, and that is adding cells.

The Recommended Dietary Allowance (RDA) for protein is 12 percent of our calories should come from protein (approximately 10 to 15 percent is fine).

Why did I tell you this? So you can be knowledgeable. So you can be suspicious of any diet low or high in protein.

Again we can be very thankful for our variety of foods, but *you need to take advantage of this variety in any diet program.* This variety is sometimes referred to as a balanced eating program. Be leery of any program that centers on a few foods, especially eating or drinking the same food twice a day.

Over the years protein has remained nearly constant at 11-12 percent of dietary energy in this country.

What's Building Your Cells Is Important

Questions you now can answer:
1. Food protein contains _____ _____.
2. All body cells contain _____.
3. Food protein's main role is to become _____
   _____.
4. The major role of dietary protein is to supply
   amino acids needed to make body _____.
5. Foods that contain all the essential amino acids
   in the correct amounts to our body's need are
   called _____ _____.
6. Non-fat or low-fat _____ _____
   are quality protein.
7. Cornbread (column 1) and beans (column 2)
   combine to make _____ _____.
8. A high protein diet may be stressful on your
   _____ and _____.
9. High protein diets cause _____ weight loss
   that is temporary.
10. Two cups of water weighs about _____ pound.
11. In any diet program we need a _____ of
    foods.

PROTEIN -   1 Gram = 4 calories ;
            1 ounce = 112 calories.
            3 to 4 hours to get into blood.
            egg (white); meat; dairy products.

FLOW CHART FOR PROTEIN AS IT ENTERS OUR BODY

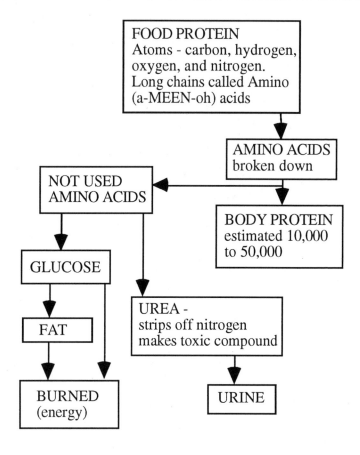

CHAPTER 9

The Wrong Thing To Eat And Why

The last body fuel is fat. It will not benefit you to know what atoms make up the compound fat. But, just as with protein and carbohydrates, it will be of great help to know the characteristics of fat and the effect it has on your body. *Fat contains nine calories per/gram and takes six to eight hours to burn.*

As a nation we have increased our consumption of fat to what some experts say is an unhealthy level. It is recommended that less than 30 percent of our calories should come from fat, yet, as a nation between 40 to 50 percent of our calories come from fat.

In 1993, based on scientific evidence, the U.S. Department of Health and Human Services reported and/or recommended the following:

1. That there is a link between diets high in fat and some cancers.
2. The Fat content of the American diet remains well above normal nutritional requirements.
3. A diet low in total fat may reduce the risk of some cancers.
4. Diets low in Saturated Fat and Cholesterol Decrease the risk of Heart Disease.
5. An easy way to reduce the levels of Saturated

Fat and Cholesterol in the diet is to reduce
total fat consumed.

6.   That less than 30 percent of your calories
should come from total fat.

The American Heart Association also recommends that less
than 30 percent of your calorie intake should come from fat.

Wouldn't it be great if every item in the grocery store stated
on the label the percent of calories that came from fat? Well,
they don't!   The government wants to recommend what's
healthy, but they don't want you to be too smart. A medical
person knows the formula to figure out the percent of calories
that come from fat, but what about the common person? With
the chart in this book, it will be easy to determine the percent
of fat. Then you can make wise choices. First, let's find out a
little more about fat.

Fats, called *lipids*, are a group of compounds that include
both fats and oils. Some fat is needed in the diet, because like
protein, it does more than just supply calories. Fat helps us
obtain the four fat-soluble vitamins, A,D,E, and K. It also
provides a long burning fuel supply, helping to keep the
body's lean tissue from being broken down for fuel.

Our body can also make fat. Even if we eat very little fat in
our diet, we can end up with fat on our body. If we eat more
calories than we burn, the extra calories will be turned into fat
and stored on our body. The body's fat mass has a virtually
unlimited storage capacity. Just what you did not want to
hear.

A person who fasts (drinking only water) will rapidly burn
body fat. *A pound of body fat will provide about 3,500
calories*. This sounds like a good way to lose weight but let's
get some more knowledge.

Fat cannot provide energy in the form of glucose. The
brain and nerves require glucose as their energy source. (Most
glucose is supplied by carbohydrates.) After a period of time
with no food coming in, the body starts to go after glucose.
The only source left for glucose is from the protein in the
muscles and other lean tissues of the body.   You need
carbohydrates daily as a source of glucose; otherwise, your
body will break down its own protein to generate glucose.
Even fat people can die from the loss of lean body tissue if
they fast too long. The message here is—variety. Once again,
the more knowledge we have about nutrition the more we see

we shouldn't starve ourselves, and we should make sure any diet has a variety of foods.

What else should you know about fat? Fat comes in three forms: *saturated fat, monounsaturated fat, and polyunsaturated fat.*

Technically they differ by the way their atoms are constructed, but let's not get that technical here. For our purposes, saturated fat is something you want to cut back on. (Approximately 10 percent of your calories should come from saturated fat.) Monounsaturated fat is OK, but polyunsaturated fat is recommended. How do you know what's what? Saturated fat is solid at room temperature, like the fat around a pork chop or lard. When you make soup or gravy and put it in the refrigerator, the fat floats to the surface and becomes hard; that's saturated fat. You would be wise to skim that off. Polyunsaturated and monounsaturated fat are both *liquid* at room temperature. Here's where you have to read the food label or look the item up in a book and know what you're looking for. If you look in a book, you may sometimes see the word "linoleic acid" for polyunsaturated fat and "oleic acid" for monounsaturated fat.

As I said, it is recommended that we increase our polyunsaturated fat and decrease our saturated fat. My dietitian recommended a ratio of at least two grams of polyunsaturated fat to one gram of saturated fat (2P:1S). When shopping for an item like margarine or mayonnaise, pick the one with the best P:S ratio if other things are equal such as cholesterol and calories.

One food with a high P:S ratio is sunflower nuts. The label states that one serving of one ounce has 10 grams of polyunsaturated fat and two grams of saturated fat. This would be written as 10:2 (meaning 10 to 2, polyunsaturated to saturated) (P:S) If we divided each number by two (factor by the smaller number), we end up with 5:1.

Although sunflower nuts have a high P:S ratio, they also derive over 70 percent of their calories from fat. This is high! My reply is—so. You need some fat in your diet, and the trick is the right kind of fat, *at the right time, and in the right amount.* Being aware of the three kinds of fat and the P:S ratio will help you eat the right kind of fat, but what's the right time?

Why would nuts or potato chips not be a good snack by themselves? Think! If you want a snack, it's because you are hungry. When you feel hungry it's because your blood sugar (glucose) is low. Will something that is mostly fat satisfy that hunger? Not for a while it won't; it takes too long to get into the bloodstream. It's not the right time. You will eat a couple of handfuls of sunflower nuts or potato chips and still be hungry so you will keep on eating. Has this ever happened to you? A good size handful is about an ounce and that's about 160 calories. Two handfuls would take up about the same space in your stomach as an apple but the apple would only be about 80 calories compared to 320 calories for the two handfuls of sunflower nuts or potato chips. The apple would go to work faster to raise your blood sugar and turn off your hunger. The amount of space a food takes up is significant because we want our stomach to feel full along with getting the right amount of calories from the right sources. It would be better to eat the apple, or another carbohydrate, and have one ounce of sunflower nuts.

One thing I do is plan my lunch so I won't be hungry later. I do this by including the sunflower nuts or almonds with my meal. The carbohydrates in my lunch will satisfy my immediate hunger, and the nuts will kick in later. The right time for a little of the right kind of fat is with carbohydrates. The nuts have what I call "staying power." (Appendix 8 lists various nuts and the amount of saturated fat.) If I should want a snack, I almost always make it a carbohydrate because it has more volume and it gets into the system faster.

I know what you are saying. I don't eat sunflower nuts and I don't snack like that. How about those potato chips? Ever check the amount of fat? You are going to eat a lot of chips before you satisfy your hunger, and we're right back to a small volume verses a large amount of calories.

How about the person who has a salad for lunch with no dressing and a bagel with no spread. They have the traditional "diet" lunch. It contains no fat. In a few hours they are hungry. Nothing they ate had any "staying power." What do they do? It's a rush to the candy machine down the hall. Sound familiar? This could have been avoided by either adding a little fat to lunch, say ten almonds or by planning for a carbohydrate snack late in the afternoon.

Remember this about fat compared to carbohydrates. *Fat usually takes up a smaller volume, gets into the system to provide energy slower, and has many more calories.* It's not the thing to eat when you are hungry.

The single most important step you can take to reduce your calorie consumption and lower cholesterol is to cut back on your fat intake. As I said, as a nation we are averaging over 40 percent of our calories from fat instead of less than 30 percent. It's obvious that overweight people could be getting well above that 40 percent figure. This is a very unhealthy but easily preventable situation.

The table below shows the grams of fat that provides between 20 and 30 percent of the calories for several total daily calorie intakes. After you determine how many calories you should be eating in a day, it is easy to select the right amount of fat. Then instead of keeping track of calories, keep track of grams of fat. Try to consume between the 20 and 30 percent figure for grams of fat.

Calories per day	Amount of fat that provides 30 % calories	Amount of fat that provides 20 % calories
1,000	33 grams	22 grams
1,500	50 grams	33 grams
2,000	67 grams	44 grams
2,500	83 grams	55 grams
3,000	100 grams	66 grams

This table appears in Appendix 18.

You don't have to deprive yourself. You do need to make some substitutions: "whole milk to non-fat milk", "butter to margarine." The only way to make wise substitutions is to read labels and be knowledgeable. If you substitute carbohydrates, for those calorie dense fats, you will be able to eat more food.

One more thing you should know about fat is the term "partially hydrogenated," because you will see it on many food labels. Hydrogenation is a chemical process where hydrogen atoms are added to unsaturated fats, making them more solid and more resistant to spoilage. This is why margarine made from vegetable oil is solid at room temperature. This process reduces the benefits of the unsaturated fat.

A HEART ATTACK CAN SAVE YOUR LIFE

Now that you know about calories, let's see how we can change what we eat (our diet) to make us healthier.

Questions you now can answer:
1. Fat contains _____ calories per gram.
2. _____ is another term for fats.
3. A pound of body fat will provide about _____ calories.
4. The three kinds of fat are _____, _____ and _____.
5. Polyunsaturated fat is _____ at room temperature.
6. When it comes to fat, it is important to eat the right kind, ____ _____ _____ and ____ _____ _____ _____.
7. Fat compared to carbohydrates, takes up less space, gets into the bloodstream _____ and has many more _____.

Bonus questions and knowledge:
According to the U.S. Department of Health and Human Services:
1. A diet low in total fat may _____ the risk of some cancers.
2. Diets low in saturated fat and cholesterol _____ the risk of Heart Disease.
3. An easy way to reduce the levels of saturated fat and cholesterol in the diet is to reduce total _____ consumed.
4. Less than ____ percent of your calories should come from fat.

FAT - 1 Gram = 9 calories;
1 ounce = 252 calories
Burns in 6 to 8 hours
Oil, butter, meats, whole milk products, cheese, potato chips, commercial products - check label.

Know the percent of calories that come from fat.

FLOW CHART FOR FAT AS IT ENTERS OUR BODY

Fat - carbon atoms with hydrogen and oxygen atoms attached.

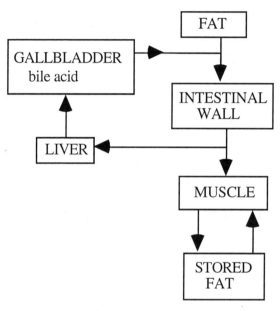

Those loaded with "H" are saturated those missing "H" are polyunsaturated.

Bile acids help digest fat. Made in the liver stored in the gallbladder.

Fat does not supply energy to brain or nervous system.

TOO MUCH MEAT MAKES THE CHURCHYARDS FAT

CHAPTER 10

The Four Letter Word Everybody Hates

The word "diet" seems to conjure up unpleasant thoughts to many people: such as eating one meal a day or eating on odd numbered days only. Many strange "FAD" diets have come and gone, because they don't work.

If you don't like the word, diet, join the crowd. Diet to me meant walking around hungry most of the day, thinking about food, and looking at the clock. I felt starved. What does the word diet mean to you? It doesn't have to be that way. Don't go on a diet. I didn't and I lost 35 pounds and they are still off. You don't need to go on a diet. You need to be knowledgeable about food and change the way you eat. It's easy once you have know-how.

According to the dictionary, diet can mean to regulate the food you eat, or it can mean a particular *selection of food*. It does not mean you starve yourself.

Many fad diets emphasize this first meaning and regulate food intake. They regulate or restrict the food so severely that you feel hungry all day. Some diets that do emphasize the selection of food make it their selection, and it may be items you don't like. How about a grapefruit with every meal? Wouldn't that get boring? Now those silly liquid diets emphasize selection—theirs; don't you think it would get boring drinking the same thing for breakfast and lunch day after day? When I think of the word, diet, I emphasize the word selection, but it should be your selection of food after you have enough knowledge to make wise choices. You should not eat food unless you like it, and you should never feel hungry.

People, at least in the United States are fortunate, we can select from a wide variety of foods. When I started to study food, I was amazed at how little most people, including me, knew about food. I had been surviving, not because of what I knew, but in spite of what I knew. I almost didn't survive my heart attack, and, if I hadn't, it would have been because of what I didn't know. When I think about that, it is downright dumb. Why do I say this? We go to school to learn a trade or profession, and we study to know the most we can about that field. Yet we won't take the time to take care of our health. Take my situation. If I had spent just a fraction of the time on nutrition that I had spent on my career, I don't think I would have had a heart attack. You don't have to go to college to study nutrition; just read a few books and follow a few basic guidelines. These guidelines have been around for a long time and are listed here.

Dietary Goals for the United States

1. To avoid being overweight, consume only as much energy (calories) as is expended; if overweight, decrease energy intake and increase energy expenditure.
2. Increase the consumption of complex carbohydrates and "naturally occurring" sugars from about 28 percent of energy intake to about 48 percent of energy intake.
3. Reduce the consumption of refined and other processed sugars by about 45 percent to account for about 10 percent of total energy intake.
4. Reduce saturated fat consumption to account for about 10 percent of total energy intake; and balance that with polyunsaturated and monounsaturated fats, which should account for about 10 percent of energy intake each.
5. Reduce cholesterol consumption to about 300 milligrams a day. (The American Heart Association has since modified this to 100 milligrams per 1,000 calories with a maximum of 300 milligrams a day.)

6. Limit the intake of sodium by reducing the intake of salt (sodium chloride) to about 5 grams a day.

Current Diet	Recommended Diet
Fat - 42%	Fat - 30%
of calories	of calories
Protein - 12%	Protein - 12%
Complex	Complex
Carbohydrate	Carbohydrate
22%	48%
Sugar - 24%	Sugar - 10%

7. *Reduce overall fat consumption from approximately 40 percent to about 30 percent of energy intake.*

Remember that these numbers are averages. Common sense should tell you that the skinny people and ideal people are below the 42 percent fat and the overweight people are above the 42 percent fat. How much above? Only taking a close look at what you eat will let you know where you stand. It wouldn't surprise me if some overweight people are getting 50-60 percent of their calories from fat, maybe more. This may kill you.

Dietary Guidelines for Americans and Suggestions for Food Choices

1. Eat a variety of foods daily. Include these foods every day: fruits and vegetables; whole grain and enriched breads and cereals; milk and milk products; meats, fish, poultry, and eggs; dried peas and beans.
2. Maintain ideal weight. Increase physical activity; reduce calories by eating fewer fatty foods and sweets and less sugar, and by avoiding too much alcohol; LOSE WEIGHT GRADUALLY.
3. Avoid too much fat, saturated fat, and cholesterol. Choose low-fat protein sources such as lean meats, fish, poultry, dried peas and beans; use eggs and organ meats in moderation; limit intake of fats on and in foods; trim fats from meats; broil, bake, or boil—don't fry; read food labels for fat contents.
4. Eat foods with adequate starch and fiber. Substitute starches for fats and sugars; select whole-grain breads and cereals, fruits and vegetables, dried beans and peas, and nuts to increase fiber and starch intake.

A HEART ATTACK CAN SAVE YOUR LIFE

5. Avoid too much sugar. Use less sugar, syrup, and honey; reduce concentrated sweets like candy, soft drinks, cookies, and the like; select fresh fruits or fruits canned in light syrup or their own juices; read food labels—sucrose, glucose, dextrose, maltose, lactose, fructose, syrups, and honey are all sugars; eat sugar less often to reduce dental caries.
6. Avoid too much sodium. Reduce salt in cooking; add little or no salt at the table; limit salty foods like potato chips, pretzels, salted nuts, popcorn, condiments, cheese, pickled foods, and cured meats; read food labels for sodium or salt contents, especially in processed and snack foods.
7. If you drink alcohol, do so in moderation. For individuals who drink—limit all alcoholic beverages (including wine, beer, liquors, and so on) to one or two drinks per day. NOTE: use of alcoholic beverages during pregnancy can result in the development of birth defects and mental retardation called Fetal Alcohol Syndrome.

The first set of seven goals is from, "Dietary Goals for the United States," 2nd ed., Select Committee on Nutrition and Human Needs, United States Senate (Washington, D.C. : Government printing Office, 1977).

The second list of seven dietary guidelines is from, "Nutrition and Your Health, Dietary Guidelines for Americans" (Washington D.C.: USDA, USDHHS, 1979).

As you can see these recommendations on how to be healthy have been around for ten years or more. It is no secret, and it's nothing new or earth shattering. The problem with Americans is, we have a quick fix mentality. We want a pill to fix our clogged arteries or to make us lose weight. We want to throw money at the problem and let someone else take care of it. We have to *learn to take charge and responsibility for our own health and eating habits.*

In the second guideline above it says, "*LOSE WEIGHT GRADUALLY.*" It has been known for a long time that losing weight too fast can cause medical problems. These problems range from heart failure and sudden death to anemia, light-headedness, constipation, gallstones, diarrhea and menstrual irregularities.

Guideline number six says, "avoid too much sodium." Why? Sodium can contribute to high blood pressure, a major risk factor for heart disease and stroke. In populations with

46

low sodium intakes, high blood pressure is rare. Excess sodium also forces your body to hold extra amounts of water. This sodium-caused edema (swelling) can cause many circulatory problems including arthritis.

Sodium is a mineral that is essential for good health; however, your body requires only a small amount, about two tenths of a gram each day. Table salt is sodium chloride—40 percent sodium. Five tenths of a gram of salt would meet your requirements for sodium, but the average American consumes between six to eighteen grams of salt daily. There are varying amounts of sodium naturally present in almost all foods, but it is not this sodium that presents the problem. It is over use of the salt shaker and sodium added during commercial processing. People who have stopped using their salt shaker think they are safe, but many sodium compounds are added during food processing. Watch food labels for soda, sodium, and the symbol Na: indicators that the product contains sodium compounds.

After reading these guidelines, you can see that you need to have a rough idea about what percentage of your calories come from fat. How else can you limit fat consumption to less than 30 percent of energy intake? That's made easy with the information in this book, and it's the key to weight and cholesterol control.

Questions you now can answer:
1. One meaning for the word, diet, is a particular
   _____ ___ _____.
2. Reduce overall fat to ____ percent or less of calorie
   intake.
3. You have to learn to _____ _____
   and _____ for your own health
   and eating habits.
4. Lose _____ gradually.

**BEING ON A DIET REQUIRES
GREAT WON'T POWER**

**IF YOU'RE LOOKING FOR
LONG-TERM HEALTH,
DON'T ACCEPT A
SHORT-TERM SOLUTION**

CHAPTER 11

It Should Be Against The Law

In March of 1990 the House of Representatives, Small Business subcommittee, conducted hearings investigating the weight-loss industry. Subcommittee chairman Rep. Ron Wyden, D-Ore., said, "Many products peddled in commercial clinics are untested, with little or no scientific proof of their safety and effectiveness." He went on to say that ". . . most experts agree that *fast weight loss is dangerous* in and of itself." One mother who testified said her 13-year-old daughter needed gallbladder surgery after a quick weight loss program. One person could not even testify because he had suffered a brain-damaging coma induced by potassium and protein deficiencies after losing nearly 35 pounds. He was a 48-year-old college engineering professor when he entered the weight loss program, and now his wife said, "He can barely summarize a Reader's Digest short article." A spokesman for the American Board of Nutrition said, "The weight-loss business in the United States has gotten out of hand." He went on to say, "The stories we've heard this morning are unfortunately all too common."

Why do smart people try rapid weight loss programs? I believe one reason is they think it must be safe or our government wouldn't let them advertise or sell the product.

Surely our government wouldn't let some company market an unsafe product or advertise something if it isn't safe, would it?

Subcommittee chairman Rep. Ron Wyden accused three federal agencies—The Food and Drug Administration, The Federal Trade Commission, and the Federal Communications Commission—of failing to ensure the safety of weight-loss products or presenting the truth of diet advertising.

In 1991 over one hundred lawsuits were filed in Dade County Florida against Nutri System. The suits alleged that the dieters were led to believe the program was safe, but that rapid weight loss without proper supervision caused them to have gallbladder disease. Many of the litigants had their gallbladders removed. The cases did not go to trial because a settlement was reached, but not discussing the settlement appears to have been one of the conditions. Who is trying to hide what? And how can the federal agencies mentioned earlier do their job if litigants are hushed up?

Let me just say, *let the buyer beware*. When it comes to your health, don't put it in anyone else's hands. Don't believe what I tell you either. Your diet, (what you eat) translates to your health and it is far too important to trust to anyone. Investigate and make it a hobby, and you will be a better person for it.

Some of the weight loss programs are expensive, if you have to buy their prepackaged foods. Do these foods have some special "keep you thin" ingredient? Why pay the high price? With a little knowledge, you can buy all the food you need right at the local supermarket to stay at an ideal weight.

Another problem diet, being advertised by celebrities, is a liquid diet. Why in the world would anyone drink two meals and eat one? You know the saying, if it walks like a duck and quacks like a duck it's probably a duck? Well, if it sounds dumb, it probably is dumb! One of my co-workers was on one of the national liquid diets at the same time I had started my new eating program. He was finished with his drink in about five minutes and I went on eating for 25 more minutes. He lost a lot of weight in one month while I only lost four pounds, but he was frustrated and cranky. He eventually put back all the weight. I just went along like a steady turtle losing a pound a week for 35 weeks. I had made some small eating habit changes that have become lifetime changes. I discovered what percent of the calories came from fat in everything I ate.

I only had to make a few changes! I wouldn't eat something that got 50 percent of it's calories from fat when something else I liked only got 10 percent of its calories from fat. I had to use a formula each time to find out what percent of the calories came from fat. You don't! All you need is the chart in this book.

The changes were easy, common sense, and good health habits. Why do I think the liquid diets are dumb? What do people do when they get to the weight they want? They do what my co-worker did. They go back to their old eating habits and right back to their old weight. He didn't know any better. He didn't increase his knowledge about food. He didn't investigate nutrition or read labels or make any lifetime changes. Wouldn't you rather eat natural foods? Don't you think natural foods are better for you? Our bodies were not designed to drink our meals.

Permanent weight control is achieved by a well-balanced, lifetime eating plan based on a variety of foods that have maximum nutritional value and not by drinking one or two meals a day. Drinking your meals sounds like a diet. Don't diet, manage your food. But you can't manage your food if you have no knowledge about food.

Here is the ultimate in "if it sounds dumb, it is." A doctor cuts you open and sucks the fat out—a procedure called liposuction. The doctor sucks out 30 pounds of fat and you weigh 30 pounds less instantly, but the very next day you are right back to your old eating habits. You will be right back to your old weight in no time. And you just blew the money for the fat suck. "No," you say, "I am going to start new habits." Then why didn't you start the new habits and lose a pound a week and save the money from the surgery for that new wardrobe? Another point is, when people are overweight, they have stored fat cells all over their body not just in the places where the doctor performs surgery. So, after the procedure, you have a fat face and a skinny waist—at least until you resume old eating habits. Sorry doctors, but this procedure just does not make sense to me, and some people have already died as a result of it. Why would anyone risk it?

Small changes in lifestyle and eating habits can save you money and will be healthier for you in the long run. Did you know if you burn an extra 100 calories a day in exercise and cut 100 calories out of your daily diet you will lose approximately 20 pounds in a year? And you will be so used to your new way of eating and living, the pounds won't ever come back. Doesn't this sound better than some of the risky diets already mentioned?

Frankly, weight reduction programs that kill people or damage their health should be against the law or at least have a warning on the label like cigarettes. Most people can't afford to have a doctor monitor their diet as closely as Oprah Winfrey did when she lost over 60 pounds in a short time. Although I never heard her promote the diet, I wonder how many viewers jumped on the bandwagon. And what happen to Oprah after her 1988 weight loss program?

Did you know that about one out of four people are on a diet of some kind? And that some diets are downright unhealthful? You should pick an eating program that is close to the guidelines mentioned earlier—approximately 12 percent protein, 30 percent fat and 58 percent carbohydrates. To be safe, lose only one-half to one pound a week, with maybe a maximum of two pounds but not for two weeks in a row. For most people it will mean cutting back on fat and increasing carbohydrates. Don't go on a diet, but manage your food. If you try the plan in this book for 37 days, you will discover how easy and safe it is to lose weight. You will love the results, and you will also get more to eat.

Questions you now can answer:
1. Most experts agree that fast weight loss is
    _____.
2. Permanent weight control is achieved by a
    _____, lifetime eating
    plan based on a _____ of foods that
    have maximum _____ value.
3. Small changes in lifestyle and eating habits
    can _____ you _____ and be
    _____ for you.

CHAPTER 12

One Good Way To Lose Weight

The original formula for healthy eating is: 4-4-2-2. This means four servings of fruits and vegetables, four servings of breads, cereals or other grains, two servings of dairy products like milk, yogurt or cheese, and two servings of lean meat, poultry, fish, or meat substitutes. A meat substitute is something that supplies the main nutrient (protein) that meat supplies, such as eggs (white), nuts or legumes. There are a few variations, but this is the basic grouping and it does provide an *acceptable foundation for meal planning*. These groups were devised based on the main *nutrient* they supply.

An updated version of this group is to separate the vegetables and fruit and include a food group for fat and put the nuts in that group. This grouping is the basis for the exchange system of food management. The exchange system was derived by a number of health organizations working with the U.S. Department of Health and Human Services. I highly recommend increasing your library and knowledge about nutrition by writing to the U.S. Department of Health and Human Services and requesting information on nutrition, exchange system, and cholesterol. You should also check with the American Dietetic Association or the American Diabetes Association, in your local telephone book, for information on the exchange system.

The exchange system sorts foods by their calories, proportions of carbohydrate, fat and protein, and portion size. Foods that are similar in nutrient content are grouped together. Therefore, any food within the group can be "exchanged" for another food within the same group, and the calories and other nutrients will be about the same. The advantage, to this system, is that it counts the calories for you. You just keep track of exchanges.

It's interesting to look at the exchange system, see how it works, and, in general, increase your knowledge about food. One of the exchange system's goals is to provide a variety of foods. So don't eat the same two fruits every day; make sure you mix them up. The exchange system is a sound basis for good meal planning, and many diet plans are based on this system.

By looking in Appendix 14, you could make different colored cards for each of the six food exchanges: fat, meat, milk, fruit, vegetables, and breads. The number of cards would represent the number of exchanges you are allowed each day. As you eat something, a card that stands for that exchange would go in a used pile, to be reused the next day. As time goes by you could write the most common things that you eat on each card. This will give you ideas of what to eat when you plan your meals. Everyone's cards will be different since our tastes vary. That's the way it should be. We are all individuals.

This sounds like Richard Simmons "Deal a Meal," which in my opinion is a spin off of the exchange system. It's a lot cheaper to make your own cards with foods you eat than to buy some expensive system. And it would be much more rewarding. You are designing a system with your new knowledge. You are making cards and writing on each card what you eat, not buying a card with something printed on it that you hate to eat. If you don't use a card system, you can use a daily log. Just mark off each exchange as you use it. Either way, it's an easy system.

Before I go on I should say, besides the "exchange system" and "Deal a Meal", "Weight Watchers" is a satisfactory program. These programs have something in common. They stress balance, variety, and slow weight loss. They reduce your fat consumption to 30 percent or less of your calories even if you don't know it. Each program has something different to offer such as meetings for support, or motivational tapes. This can be expensive. One months fee can easily be more than this book.

This book is designed to give you the knowledge to eat healthy, lose weight, and reduce cholesterol. But don't trust any program by following it blindly, not even mine. Check out claims and statements with reference books in the library or with your doctor.

The table that follows shows the number of exchanges for various calorie intakes. You should have the number of cards equal to the exchanges for your calories. The number of calories in one exchange is in parenthesis. To see a listing of foods in each exchange turn to Appendix 14. Milk and meat items are high in fat, so they not only count as an exchange in their group but, they also count as a fat exchange. This is noted in Appendix 14.

	CALORIES per/day				
Exchanges	1,000	1,200	1,500	1,800	2,000
Bread (70)	4	5	8	10	10
Vegetable (25)	2	3	3	3	4
Fruit (40)	3	4	4	5	5
Milk (80)	2	2	2	2	3
Lean Meat (55)	4	5	5	6	7
Fat (45)	4	5	6	7	8

The above table will supply about 30 percent of your total calories from fat. The fat contained in lean meat was taken into account; any other meat will decrease your fat exchanges.

How do you use this chart? If you decide you should have 1,500 calories per/day find 1,500 on the chart and go straight down. The first number you run into is eight which is across from bread; you are allowed eight bread exchanges. The next number is three across from vegetables, four across from fruit, two milk, five meat, and six fat. This is a total of 28 exchanges to be used each day. To see what constitutes one exchange look in Appendix 14.

You will notice that a person who should be getting 2,000 calories, such as myself, would be allowed seven lean meat exchanges. This means about seven ounces of meat per/day. One meat exchange is equal to one ounce of lean meat. I usually have less because I am trying to keep my cholesterol down. Some experts suggest that six ounces of meat should be the maximum. Remember these are just guidelines, nothing hard and fast. You could reduce the meat and fat exchanges and increase the others; this would decrease the percent of your calories that come from fat. *Your goal should be an ideal weight and an ideal blood cholesterol level.*

To figure out how many exchanges you're allowed, you first have to know how many calories you should be getting if you want to lose weight. The most accurate way to do this is to figure out how many calories you are getting right now, and then reduce that amount by 200 to 500 calories but no more. You want to end up losing a half to one pound a week and change to good eating habits.

A second system is the one my dietitian gave me. Look up your ideal weight and multiply by 10, this is the calorie intake to lose weight for men. Mine was 140 pounds times 10, or 1,400 calories per/day. When you reach your ideal weight multiply it by 15, this is your new calorie intake to maintain that weight. Mine is 140 pounds times 15, or 2,100 calories. Women will have to subtract about 200 to 400 calories from the figure they come up with. Remember, this second system is just a rule of thumb and may not work for everyone. In fact, mine was on the low side. You will notice the difference is 700 calories. Many weeks I lost two pounds. With what I have learned since then, I realize I probably should have been eating about 1,800 calories to lose weight more slowly. The only sure way to find out just how many calories you are eating now is to write down what you eat, and then you will have a basis for making changes.

What I did was a little different from the exchange system because I wrote down everything I ate. I was concerned with my calories and my cholesterol intake. I planned my meals around the cholesterol level of the foods I ate. I tried not to go over 200 Mg. of cholesterol in a day. This meant I had to fill in around the cholesterol food with fruits, vegetables, and breads. This really worked out to be very close to the exchange system, before I even knew about it. I made drastic changes because I had already had a heart attack. You may only need to make minor changes. I cannot over emphasize that we are all individuals. We won't all be eating the same thing or doing the same exercise. What you do depends on: age, sex, heart condition, weight, and cholesterol levels. The information is here to set up a program that will make you healthier.

In a later chapter, I provide a sample of how to list things to eat for breakfast, lunch, and supper. Add your items to these lists and keep in mind the exchange system; plan your meals using these lists. It is important when using the exchange system not to go over the limits for fat or meat. You want this to be a habit forming program that you can follow for the rest of your life. Remember, you're not going on a diet, but changing the way you eat. In fact, you will get more to eat.

Here Are Some Other
Things to Consider

Your current eating habits took years to develop. Don't panic if you start a program and slip; we all do. I still put salt on my popcorn. In fact, I have what I call a party day once or twice a week, where I eat foods that aren't the best. The difference is I plan for these days; I don't feel guilty or that I'm cheating. I know the percent of fat in everything I eat. Keep at it until you find a plan that works for you. Learn all you can about the foods you eat.

Don't Skip Meals!
Don't Go Hungry!

Learn to take your time eating. *It takes your brain about 20 minutes to let you know you're full.*

As you add foods to the exchange list or meal list, watch for items high in fat content. *Calories from fat are more likely to end up as fat on your body than calories from protein or carbohydrates.* Add complex carbohydrates to your meals and snacks. Endurance athletes know the value of complex carbohydrates.

Learn to Read Labels and
Watch for Hidden Fats

Watch the fast food restaurants. A hamburger, fries, and shake will be over 30 grams of fat and 800 plus calories. Many restaurants, like McDonald's, will supply you with nutrition information if you ask. Many of these restaurants now have low fat items, but take the time to check out the fat content yourself.

Percent of Calories from Fat

Use the charts in this book to determine the percent of calories that come from fat. Everyone should know what percent of calories come from fat in everything they eat. I don't think you can lose weight and keep it off if more than 30 percent of your calories come from fat. It's not like you'll be looking things up all the time. Once you check something out, you'll remember whether it's something you can have any time or just once in a while.

Avoid fad diets and rapid weight loss.

Most of the weight loss is water and will come right back. Most people regain the weight plus some. Beware of low calorie diets and those centered on a few foods. You need a *variety* of foods and enough calories to assure you will be getting all the *nutrients* you need. Be suspicious of large weight loss claims. My claim is, if you follow the guidelines in this book you will lose a half to one pound a week. That's 26 to 52 pounds in a year. If you lose more, please increase what you are eating but make it complex carbohydrates.

Plan Each Meal

Put some real thought behind it. Remember the information about protein? What foods do you combine to get a complete protein? Go back and read the section on protein and tear out that appendix and post it right on the refrigerator. When I started my program, once a week I would plan the dinner meals for that week. I tried to include one fish meal and one meatless meal a week. You need to learn to plan your meals.

One Good Way To Lose Weight

Questions you now can answer:
1. The exchange system does provide an _____
   _____ for meal planning.
2. The exchange system groups foods by the main
   _____ they supply.
3. Your goal should be an _____ _____
   and an _____ _____ _____
4. It takes your brain _____
   _____ . So eat slowly.
5. _____ _____ _____ are more likely
   to end up as fat on your body than calories from
   protein or carbohydrates.
6. Avoid fad_____ and rapid _____ loss.
7. You need a _____ of foods and enough
   calories to assure you will be getting all the
   _____ you need.

ONLY ONE PERSON

CAN DEFEAT YOU

CHAPTER 13

How To Discover What's In It

Food labels have become scorecards for millions of health-conscious Americans. And with good reason; for today food labels contain a wealth of information.

Facts found on labels tell not only what the product is, but also they may tell what ingredients are in it, the nutrient value of those ingredients, the company responsible for the product, and, frequently, the date by which it should be sold.

Furthermore, labels may give details about substances that a person wishes to avoid, such as fat, sodium, or cholesterol. Indeed, Food and Drug Administration, (FDA) surveys show that about four out of five people look at the ingredients. More than two out of three people say they're looking at labels for substances they want to avoid for health reasons.

The amount of information on food labels varies, but all food labels must contain at least the following:

    * the name of the product,
    * the net contents or net weight, which includes the
       liquid in canned foods, and
    * the name and place of business of the manufacturer,
       packer or distributor.

Here's a rundown on some of the other information that may be found on food labels:

1. List of Ingredients

For most foods, all of the ingredients must be listed on the label and must be identified by their common or usual names. The ingredient that is present in the largest amount, by weight, *must be listed first,* with the other ingredients following in descending order according to weight.

Any additives must also be listed. If colors and flavors are used, the law permits the use of such general language as "artificial color," "artificial flavor," or "natural flavor." (The only exception to the rule about artificial colors is their use in butter, cheese, and ice cream.) However, the use of the color Yellow No. 5 must be identified specifically in all products because it can cause allergic reactions in some persons.

2. Nutrition Information

Nutrition information is required on a food label when a manufacturer adds a nutrient to it or when a claim is made for the product, such as "now contains fewer calories." Protein and certain vitamins and minerals may be added by manufacturers to make a food more nutritious or to restore nutrients lost in processing.

Many food products don't require nutrition labeling, but the manufacturers include the information anyway, knowing how important nutrition information is to consumers. Indeed, better than half the processed foods found in stores contain labeling with nutritional information. On the next page is an example of a nutrition label.

Nutrition Information Per Serving
Serving size = one-half cup
Servings per container = 12
Calories   190
Protein   2 grams
Carbohydrate   24 grams
Fat   9 grams
Sodium   55 milligrams
Percentage of U.S. Recommended Daily
Allowances (U.S. RDA)*
Protein   4
Thiamine   10
Niacin   2

*Contains less than 2 percent of the U.S. RDA of vitamin A, vitamin C, riboflavin, calcium and iron.
(Note: There are 28.35 grams per ounce, and 1,000 milligrams in a gram.)
Note that the top part gives the number of calories and the amount of protein, carbohydrates, fat and sodium—in that order—in a specified serving of the product. Manufacturers also have the option of listing cholesterol, fatty acids, and potassium content.

The following was taken from, "The New Food Label Summaries" a booklet available through the Food and Drug Administration, 200 C St. SW, Washington DC 20204.
This Labeling became effective May 8, 1994
==
Mandatory Nutrition Labeling
Brief Summary: FDA is amending its regulations to require nutrition labeling for most foods offered for sale and regulated by FDA. The nutrition label is required to include information on total calories and calories from fat and on amounts of total fat, saturated fat, cholesterol, sodium, total carbohydrates, dietary fiber, sugars, protein, vitamin A, vitamin C, calcium, and iron — in that order. Manufacturers also may voluntarily declare information on calories from saturated fat and on amounts of polyunsaturated and monounsaturated fat, soluble and insoluble fiber, sugar alcohol, other carbohydrate, potassium, additional vitamins and minerals for which Reference Daily Intakes (RDIs) have been established, and the percent of vitamin A present as beta-carotene. The information

presented on the label is to represent the packaged product prior to consumer preparation.

This final rule establishes a standard format for nutrition information on food labels consisting of:

1. the quantitative amount per serving of each nutrient except vitamins and minerals;
2. the amount of each nutrient as a percent of the Daily Value for a 2,000 calorie diet
3. a footnote with reference values for selected nutrients based on 2,000 calorie and 2,500 calorie diets; and
4. caloric conversion information.

The declaration of percent of Daily Value must be placed in column order. Absolute declarations of the amount per serving of designated nutrients must appear immediately following the nutrient named. A simplified format may be used if seven or more of 13 required nutrients are present in only insignificant amounts.

Foods exempt from mandatory nutrition labeling requirements include:

1. food offered for sale by small businesses;
2. food sold in restaurants or other establishments in which food is served for immediate human consumption;
3. foods similar to restaurant foods that are ready to eat but are not for immediate consumption, are primarily prepared on site, and are not offered for sale outside of that location;
4. foods that contain insignificant amounts of all nutrients subject to this rule, e.g., coffee and tea;
5. dietary supplements, except those in conventional food form;
6. infant formula;
7. medical foods;
8. custom-processed fish or game meats;
9. foods shipped in bulk form; and
10. donated foods. Otherwise-exempted foods that make a nutrient content claim or health claim forfeit the exemption.

Special labeling provisions specify that:

1. foods in small packages having less than 12 square inches available for labeling may omit nutrition labeling if an address or telephone number that a consumer may use to obtain required nutrition information is provided on the label;

2. packages of 40 or fewer square inches may present the required information in tabular or linear fashion if the package shape cannot accommodate columns, use specified abbreviations, omit the footnote and caloric conversion information, and present the required nutrition information on any label panel;

3. foods for children less than two years of age must not declare information concerning calories from fat, fatty acids and cholesterol;

4. foods for children less than four years of age must not include Daily Value information;

5. raw fruits, vegetables, and fish should follow voluntary nutrition labeling guidelines;

6. packaged single-ingredient fish or game meat may provide information on an "as prepared" basis;

7. foods sold from bulk containers and game meat products may provide nutrition information on labeling;

8. shell eggs may provide the required nutrition information inside the egg carton;

9. under certain conditions, unit containers in multi-unit packages need only provide nutrition information on the outer package; and

10. foods in gift packs may provide information on labeling in accordance with special requirements.

A standard format label would look like this:

       Nutrition Facts
       Serving Size 1/2 cup (114g)
       Servings per container 4
       Amount Per Serving
       Calories 260 Calories from fat 120

% Daily value*

Total Fat 13 g	20%
Saturated Fat 5 g	25%
Cholesterol 30 mg	10%
Sodium 660 mg	28%
Total Carbohydrate 31 g	11%
Dietary Fiber 0 g	0%

Sugars 5 g
Protein 5g
Vitamin A 4%   Vitamin C 2%
Calcium 15% Iron 4%

* Percent Daily Values are based on a 2,000 calorie diet. Your daily values may be higher or lower depending on your calorie needs:

Nutrient	2,000 Calories	2,500 Calories
Total Fat less than	65g	80g
Sat Fat less than	20g	25g
Cholesterol less than	300mg	300mg
Sodium—less than	2,400mg	2,400mg
Total Carbohydrate	300g	375g
Fiber	25g	30g

Calories per gram:
Fat 9 - Carbohydrates 4 - Protein 4

Reference Daily Intakes and Reference Values

Brief Summary: This regulation establishes reference values for use in nutrition labeling of food. It retains the values established by FDA in 1973 for vitamins and minerals but changes the terms for those values from U.S. Recommended Daily Allowance (U.S. RDA) to Reference Daily Intake (RDI). The regulation also establishes label reference values for eight other nutrients, including fat, cholesterol, and fiber. The values have been established as Daily Reference Values (DRVs). While regulatory requirements make it necessary to distinguish between the two sets of label reference values, to avoid needless confusion, all reference values on food labels will be referred to as Daily Values or DVs.

FDA received more than 1,500 written comments on its proposals published in July 1990 and November 1991 to revise and expand U.S.RDAs to be consistent with the 1989 edition of the Recommended Daily Allowances established by the National Academy of Sciences, and to develop new label reference values for nutrients important to health but for which the Academy had not established RDAs. These comments offered suggestions for changes, but generally supported FDA's efforts to update label reference values for vitamins and minerals and create new values for nutrients of public health importance.

On October 29, 1992, the Dietary Supplement Act of 1992 was signed into law. The act, among other provisions, instructed FDA to not promulgate regulations prior to November 8, 1993 that require the use of, or are based on, RDAs for vitamins and minerals. In effect, the Act required FDA to retain current U.S.RDA values for vitamins and minerals, values that had been developed chiefly by selecting the highest RDA value from among the various sex/age groups listed in RDA tables published in 1968.

Accordingly, this final rule establishes label reference values for 19 vitamins and minerals that are the same as those in existing regulations and that are appropriate for use on foods intended for adults and children four or more years of age. These values, however, will no longer be called U.S.RDAs, but instead will be known as RDIs, a change the Agency agrees is necessary to minimize confusion between RDAs and U.S.RDAs. Since the Dietary Supplement Act did not provide for reference values for infants, children less than four years of age, pregnant women, and lactating women, the preamble to this final rule includes guidance on values that manufacturers may use on labels intended for those groups.

Additionally, the Agency established Daily Reference Values for other nutrients of public health importance which are intended to serve as a point of reference for adults and children four or more years of age. When appropriate, a caloric intake of 2,000 calories per day was used as the basis for these reference values. The nutrients with DRVs are: fat (65 grams), saturated fat (20 grams), cholesterol (300 milligrams), total

carbohydrate (300 grams), dietary fiber (25 grams), sodium (2,400 milligrams), potassium (3,500 milligrams), and protein (50 grams).
= =
All of the proceeding came from the booklet "The New Food Label Summaries".

The new label has one glaring flaw. The percentages for daily values are based on 2,000 calories. If your calorie needs are above or below 2,000 then these percentages do not apply to you. Did the government forget we are individuals? How many women consume less than 2,000 calories a day? Who came up with the magic number of 2,000 calories, a man? The fact is, if you are a 1,500 calorie person the new labels "Percent Daily Value" for total fat will actually put you over the recommended 30 percent of calories from fat.

Here's how that would work comparing a 2,000 calorie person to a 1,500 calorie person.

A 2,000 calorie person who adds up the percent Daily Value for fat could eat five items like our sample label, each one is 20% fat. (20% x 5 = 100%) They could then eat zero fat items until their total calories were 2,000.

> Their result: 2,000 total calories; 600 calories
> from fat (120 x 5 = 600)
> To figure their % of calories from fat divide
> fat calories by total calories
> or 600 divided by 2,000 = 30%

A 1,500 calorie person who mistakenly thinks they can just add % Daily Value for fat until they get to 100% would look like this. Five similar items for 100% fat and 600 calories, zero fat items until their total calories were up to 1,500.

> Their result: 1,500 total calories; 600 calories
> from fat (120 x 5 = 600)
> To figure their % of calories from fat divide
> fat calories by total calories
> or 600 divided by 1,500 = 40%

The moral? Is the "Percent Daily Value" for fat of much use to a 1,500 calorie person?

What would be more beneficial to everyone on the new labels? What's missing from the old and new labels? Isn't it the recommendation of nutrition experts, including the U.S.

Government, that we obtain less than 30 percent of our total calories from fat? Don't you think it's strange that our government has known for over ten years that to be healthy we should obtain less than thirty percent of our calories from fat—yet this simple figure is not required on food labels? Can you readily tell the percent of calories from fat on this label? Of course not. In fact some labels are misleading, and I will discuss these later. You can't read the percent of calories from fat directly, but you can figure it out with the information listed if you do a little math.

Remember there are nine calories in one gram of fat. Multiply nine calories by the thirteen grams of listed fat, on the previous label, for a total of one hundred and seventeen ($9 \times 13 = 117$). (NOTE: The label lists 120 as calories from fat and not 117. Manufacturers are given some flexibility to round off their data and still be in accordance with government regulations.) Then divide the 117 by the total calories of 260. (117 divided by 260 = .45 or 45 percent) This means 45 percent of the calories come from fat. This figure is not required on food labels. Weight Watchers knows the importance of letting the consumer know the percent of calories from fat and voluntarily puts that information on their products. Thanks Weight Watchers for knowing what weight conscious and health conscious consumers need even if the FDA doesn't.

Most people don't want to do math problems in the grocery store. At the end of this chapter is a chart that you can use to quickly find the percent of calories from fat. The chart also appears in Appendix 17. This is valuable information in comparing similar products.

Questions you now can answer:
1. The ingredient that is present in the largest amount, by weight, _____ ____ _____ _____.
2. The percent of Daily Values listed on new food labels is based on _____ calories.

E-Z-2 READ
PERCENT OF CALORIES FROM FAT CHART

Find the calories and grams of FAT per serving. Where the values intersect is how much of the serving is FAT. For example: 110 calories and 5 grams of fat = 41 % FAT.

FAT grams	1	2	3	4	5	6	7	8	9	10	11
CALORIES											
60	15	30	45	60	75	90	**	**	**	**	**
70	13	26	39	51	64	77	90	**	**	**	**
80	11	23	34	45	56	68	79	90	**	**	**
90	10	20	30	40	50	60	70	80	90	**	**
100	9	18	27	36	45	54	63	72	81	90	**
110	8	16	25	33	41	49	57	65	74	82	90
120	8	15	23	30	38	45	53	60	68	75	83
130	7	14	21	28	35	42	48	55	62	69	76
140	6	13	19	26	32	39	45	51	58	64	71
150	6	12	18	24	30	36	42	48	54	60	66
200	5	9	14	18	23	27	32	36	41	45	50
250	4	7	11	14	18	22	25	29	32	36	40
300	3	6	9	12	15	18	21	24	27	30	33
350	3	5	8	10	13	15	18	21	23	26	28
400	2	5	7	9	11	14	16	18	20	23	25

** = Over 90 percent fat.

It is recommended that no more than 30 percent of your total calories come from fat.

NOTE: If you had numbers not on the chart, such as 500 calories and 20 grams of fat, you could divide each number by the same number to get back on the chart.

ORDER FROM: READERS CHOICE, 2141 Shaw Ave., Suite 1212, Clovis, CA. 93611-8916

$1 for plastic wallet size - plus self-addressed stamped envelope please. Great for the grocery store.

$3 for a magnetic-back chart that mounts on refrigerator size (4" by 6") - plus self-addressed stamped (2 ounces postage) and #10 envelope please.

CHAPTER 14

Moderation - Mom Was Right

I was introduced to reading food labels during my rehabilitation course after my heart attack. I knew some foods had food labels, but I didn't pay much attention to them. I really wouldn't have known what I was looking for anyway. The dietitian teaching the class said that if we wanted to take charge of our health, we had to start reading and understanding food labels.

It was while taking these courses that I decided to write down what I ate. As I started to do this, I found that many of the foods I ate did not list the protein, carbohydrates, and fat. I made the decision not to eat processed foods that did not list these items. I felt that if the manufacturers would not tell me how much fat was in their product, I wouldn't eat it. What are the manufacturers hiding anyway? Since that time, many more companies have started to list the amount of protein, carbohydrates, and fat.

I also wrote to many companies and tried to find out how much fat and cholesterol was in their products. Some companies responded with the information I requested. If you are interested, you should do the same thing. Other companies were evasive and those products I no longer buy or eat.

Some companies say they may use any one of a number of oils in their product. They state they may use palm oil, coconut oil, or safflower oil and you don't know which. Each batch of their product may contain a different oil. It probably just depends on which is the cheapest oil at the time. This might not be so bad if some of these oils weren't bad for our hearts and if they didn't clog our arteries. Take a look at Appendix 7 and you can see the difference in these oils.

One of the products recommended by my dietitian was Hollywood Oil. They have two oils on the market, Canola and Safflower. Canola oil is high in monounsaturated fat while Safflower oil is high in polyunsaturated fat; yet both are low in saturated fat. I use these oils in recipes and I have a few salad dressings I make with these oils. Of course you realize that all the calories in oil come from fat.

Let's take a look at a few food labels.

SAMPLE PRODUCT LABELS

Multi-Bran Chex made by Ralston Purina Company

Serving size - 2/3 Cup

Calories	90	
Protein	2	gram
Carbohydrate	25	gram
Fat	0	gram
Cholesterol	0	mg
Sodium	200	mg

Carbohydrate Information

Starch & related
Carbohydrates ------- 15 grams
Sucrose & other
Sugars ----------------- 6 grams
Dietary Fiber --------- 4 grams

Total
Carbohydrates ---------------- 25 grams

As you can see, there is no cholesterol and no fat. Also the manufacturer has broken down the carbohydrates so that you can see the amount of complex carbohydrates. Try this or another wholesome cereal as a snack instead of potato chips with your lunch.

Total Raisin Bran by General Mills

> Serving size 1.5 ounces
> Calories ------------- 140
> Protein ----------------- 3 gram
> Carbohydrate --------- 33 gram
> Fat ---------------------- 1 gram
> Cholesterol ------------ 0 mg
> Sodium -------------- 190 mg
> Potassium ----------- 220 mg

Carbohydrate Information

> Complex
> Carbohydrates ------- 19grams
> Sucrose & other
> Sugars ** ------------ 14 grams
> Dietary Fiber ---------- 5 grams
> Total   _____

Carbohydrates ----------------- 33 grams

** 9 of the 14 grams of sugar occur naturally in raisins. (The manufacturer wants you to know that most of the sugar is natural.)

The cells of your brain and nervous system depend on sugar for their energy. The best source of sugar is fruit.

Here's a look at a couple of lunch meat labels.

Oscar Mayer Ham versus Beef Bologna

	HAM	BOLOGNA
Serving size	1 Slice	1 Slice
Calories	20	90
Protein	4 gram	3 gram
Carbohydrate	*	1 gram
Fat	*	8 gram
Cholesterol	10 mg	20 mg
Sodium	280 mg	310 mg

* Contains less than 1 gram.

The Bologna gets 80 percent of the calories from fat. Which one should you choose for lunch? It's not hard to make the right choice once you know what you're looking for.

Now here's one item that I won't recommend; it's a snack cracker. I used to take this in my lunch quite often prior to my heart attack.

Serving size - (about 1/2 ounce)
Calories -------------70
Protein ---------------2 gram
Carbohydrate --------7 gram
Fat --------------------4 gram
Polyunsaturated------ *
Saturated ------------- 1 gram
Cholesterol less than --------2 mg
Sodium ------------ 135 mg

* Contains less than 1 gram.

The Ingredients list states ". . .Vegetable Shortening (contains one or more of the following partially hydrogenated oils: Soybean, Cottonseed, Canola). . ."

Based on the four grams of fat times nine, (36) divided by 70 calories, we have 51 percent of the calories from fat. (see chart at the end of the previous chapter)

On this box of crackers it also says "Low Cholesterol," which it is, and "contains 100% natural cheese made from skim milk." These are just come-ons. Too bad it doesn't say 51 percent of the calories come from fat. In fact, it wouldn't be a bad idea if the percent of calories from fat were required to be on every label.

Don't get me wrong, I still eat this cracker but very infrequently. I put it in with the group of foods that include such items as ice cream, which, are high in fat and should be eaten less often. This is just what you need to do. Investigate all the foods you eat. Know what's in them and decide if you should cut back or switch to something you like equally well that contains less fat. I used to eat ice cream a lot. I satisfy that urge with a fudge bar that has no fat and I have ice cream only occasionally.

It is important to note that most of the calories in the fudge bar come from sugar. It is not something that should scare you off of them, but you shouldn't be eating three or four a day either.

Pretzels and bagels or bagel chips have about 100 to 150 calories in a serving and one gram of fat. They are below 10 percent fat. They are a great substitute for potato chips or corn chips which run over 50 percent fat. Check it out.

These are the kinds of changes a person can make when one gets used to looking at labels. The key is to be knowledgeable.

"Moderation," my mother used to say, "everything in moderation." Yes, but without knowledge about what is in various foods, how do you know what to moderate? How do you know that one item is 15 percent fat and another 60 percent fat? These may be foods that you like equally well, and if you were knowledgeable, you would make the wise choice.

What does it mean if something, say a cookie, is 50 percent fat? It means, in terms of calories, that half of the cookie is made up of fat and the other half is made up of all the other ingredients: flour, sugar, baking soda. Imagine that cookie on a plate. Take a long hard look. Visualize half of that cookie as fat! Would you eat the fat that bacon floats in? That's what you are going to do when you eat that cookie or any other high fat item. Many snacks are over 50 percent fat. You can not lose weight, or reduce heart attack and cancer risks until you get a handle on these high fat items. You must know the percent of fat in everything you eat so you can make wise choices. Use the "Percent of Calories from Fat Chart."

Before I go on, let me mention one more product I use—Egg Beaters. Here is a comparison of this egg substitute to a real egg.

	Egg Beaters	Real Egg
Calories	25	70
Protein, grams	5	5
Carbohydrate	1 gram	1 gram
Fat	0 gram	5 gram
CHOLESTEROL	0 mg.	240 mg.
Sodium	80 mg.	60 mg.

Egg Beaters is 99 percent real egg white. Egg white and non-fat milk are very good sources of protein.

SUMMARY:
1. Learn to read labels.
2. Know the percent of calories that come from fat in everything you eat. Use the chart in the last chapter.
3. Slowly shift to foods that are better for you: ones that have less fat and cholesterol.
4. Plan all meals.

THE BEST
HEALTH INSURANCE
IS
MODERATION

CHAPTER 15

97 % Fat Free - What You Should Know

The part of the food label discussed so far is factual and of value to the consumer. It is also in the smallest print. What's in large print is another matter.

"NO CHOLESTEROL" and "NO FAT" are also factual and of value but in many cases obvious.

The problem lies in the phrase "97% FAT FREE" usually written in very large letters. Just what does "97 PERCENT FAT FREE" mean? From this label can you tell what percent of calories come from fat? *Of course not.*

Here's how that "97% FAT FREE" works. The three nutrients, protein, carbohydrates, and fat are listed on a food label along with how many grams are in a serving. One would think that if you add the weight of the protein, carbohydrates, and fat you would come up with the total weight of the product. This will not be the case. In some products there will be quite a discrepancy between the weight of the product and the total weight of the three listed nutrients. The missing nutrient is water.

By law, the percent of nutrients on food labels is listed as percent by weight, not percent by calories, which would be more helpful. In this way the manufacturer is comparing the *fat weight to the total weight,* which includes those items that do not contribute calories. This percentage is then displayed on the label. If a manufacturer has a product that's only 50 percent fat free by weight and wants to make it 80 percent fat free, *water* is just added.

Don't get me wrong! You can still benefit from this type of label but not as much as you could if manufacturers were required to list the percent of calories from fat. We should all write to the Department of Health and Human Services, and express our concern that food labels contain the percent of calories from fat information that is vital for good health. See the sample letter at the end of this chapter.

Take the hot dog whose label states 80 percent fat free. It probably contains a lower percent of calories from fat than the regular hot dogs, but the only way to know for sure is to figure it out. The "Percent of Calories from Fat Chart" will aid you in computing this information. (see Appendix 17)

Let's take a look at the wrapper of Oscar Mayer Light Beef Franks:

     1/3 less fat*
     80% FAT FREE
     20% FAT

* This product contains no more than 20% Fat which is 33% less fat than the USDA standard.

Isn't all this information confusing to the consumer? What are all these percentages? All you need to know are the total calories in a serving, which are 130, and the total grams of fat in a serving, which are 11, and with the previous chart you see 76 percent of the calories come from fat. If you knew this you might choose a different type of meat. But you can't determine this, at least not easily, so do you have a choice?

Here's the entire Oscar Mayer label:
OSCAR MAYER - Light Beef Franks
       1/3 less Fat   80% Fat Free 20% Fat
       Net Wt. 16 oz. (1 pound) 454 grams
       Portion size 1 link (57 grams)
              Portions Per Container 8
              Calories   130
              Protein --------------- 7 -- grams
              Carbohydrate -------- 1 -- gram
              Fat -------------------- 11 -- grams
              TOTAL -------------- 19 -- grams Per serving

It would appear that the weight of one serving is 19 grams but let's not assume anything. If we multiply the 19 grams,(weight of one serving) by the 8 servings, we get 152 grams, the total for the whole package. But the manufacturer has already stated there are 454 grams (1 pound) in this package. How did we lose 302 grams? (454 minus 152 equals 302) Over half the weight is not accounted for in protein, carbohydrates, or fat. So what happened to the 302 missing grams? The missing weight has to be somewhere in the list of ingredients.

<u>Ingredients</u>: Beef, WATER, Salt, Corn Syrup, Dextrose, Hydrolyzed Milk Protein, Flavoring, Sodium Phosphates, Sodium erythorbate, Extractives of Paprika, Sodium Nitrite.

As you can see, the second ingredient is water and this accounts for most of the lost weight which isn't clearly reported.

It would be much more meaningful if manufacturers placed the number of calories and the percent this represented of the total calories next to the weight for protein, carbohydrates, and fat. Our hot dogs would then look like this:

Total Calories 130

Protein	7 grams	28 Calories	21%
Carbohydrates	1gram	4 Calories	3%
Fat	11 grams	99 Calories	76%

Wouldn't this be much more meaningful and useful to the consumer?

In contrast take a look at Nabisco Wheat Thins:

> Net Weight 16 oz. (1 Pound) 454 grams
> Serving Size 1/2 ounce (8 crackers)
> Servings Per Package 32
> Calories 70
>
> | Protein | 1 | gram |
> |---|---|---|
> | Carbohydrates | 9 | grams |
> | Fat | 3 | grams |
> | Total | 13 | grams Per Serving |

The 13 grams per serving times 32 servings equals 416 total grams. When you subtract the 416 grams from 454 total grams, you end up with 38 missing grams. Much better than the 302 grams missing in the hot dogs.

Also using the "Percent of Fat Chart," you can see that 39 percent of the calories come from fat. (Find 70 calories and three grams of fat on the chart.) This is a much better snack than potato chips or corn chips which are over 50 percent fat. You won't lose weight eating those chips.

My kids like graham crackers and so do I. There are several brands to choose from. Most have 60 calories in a serving, but Nabisco has only one gram of fat while the others have three grams of fat. That means Nabisco graham crackers are 15 percent fat while the others are 45 percent fat. That's the kind of information I hope you will gain from this book.

One more product I'd like to mention is Nabisco Fat Free Premium Crackers:

Net Wt. 15 oz. 425 grams

> Serving Size 1/2 oz.
> Servings Per Package 30
>
> | Protein | 1 | gram |
> |---|---|---|
> | Carbohydrate | 12 | grams |
> | Fat | 0 | grams |
> | Total | 13 | grams Per Serving |

As I said earlier if the label states "Fat Free," you can feel fairly certain that it is, but check the small print anyway. In this case, it is fat free.

Nabisco appears to be the leader in no fat contents or reducing the fat in their cookie and snack products.

The meats, poultry, and fish I have listed in the appendix show the percentage of calories from fat.

97 % Fat Free - What You Should Know

Questions you now can answer:
1. If a food label says, "97 % Fat Free," can you tell what percent of the calories come from fat?_____ _____ _____.

2. The manufacturer is comparing the _____ _____ to the total _____.

3. If a manufacturer has a product that's 50 percent fat free and would like to make it 80 percent fat free _____ is just added.

A HEART ATTACK CAN SAVE YOUR LIFE

Department of Health and Human Services
Food and Drug Administration
5600 Fishers Lane
Rockville, Md. 20857

Dear Sir:

I wish to comment on the "New Nutrition Labeling". In order to identify the most healthful foods, it would be extremely helpful if the percent of calories that come from protein, carbohydrates, and fat were listed. A typical label follows, only I've put what should also be added to the label in parenthesis.

			ADD BELOW
Total Calories	130		
Protein	7	grams	(28 calories 21 %)
Carbohydrates	1	gram	(4 calories 3 %)
Fat	11	grams	(99 calories 76 %)

This is an actual label minus what's in parenthesis. On the front of the label it states "80 % FAT FREE." This is because under current rules, the manufacturer compares the fat in the product to the total weight of the product. In this case the weight has been increased by the addition of water. As long as the U.S. Government recommends that we obtain no more than 30 percent of our calories from fat it would make sense that this information would be readily available. If we knew the percent of calories that came from fat we could make more healthful choices.

A newspaper article stated . . . "FDA officials said they have estimated that the regulations will lead to such improved eating habits that 39,000 cases of cancer and heart disease will be prevented over the next 20 years and health-care expenditures will be cut by $100 billion."

As a heart patient and tax payer this would be good news but only if the new labels provide the consumers with meaningful information. I want to look at a label and know right away what percent of the calories come from fat.
                    Sincerely,

CHAPTER 16

The Secret to Permanent Weight Control

Ever say, "How can Jane or Dick eat so much and stay so thin?" We have all known people who ate a lot and stayed thin. We may have heard their metabolism was high but what does that mean exactly?

Did you ever lose a lot of weight in a short time or know someone who did only to regain it all like Oprah Winfrey? The answer may be in understanding how your metabolism works.

In earlier chapters I discussed where calories come from and how they function as our energy source. How are these calories used? Exercise? Surprisingly, to most people, very few calories are used during exercise.

Calories are used in three ways:
1. Digesting food
2. Physical Activity
3. Basal Metabolic Rate (BMR)

The percentage of your total calories, each of these uses, remains fairly constant: *digestion 10 percent, physical activity*

25 percent, and basal metabolic rate 65 percent. While you can't change the percent each of these uses, you can change your calorie demand, and thus, alter the total calories required by your body. A person who consumes 1,000 calories a day uses 10 percent or 100 calories to digest that food, and a person who consumes 3,000 calories uses 10 percent or 300 calories to digest that food. While digestion stayed at 10 percent, the calories used to burn the food you ate increased from 100 to 300 by eating more. You need to find an area where you will burn more calories without eating more.

The second use of calories is physical activity—all physical activity. Getting up out of your chair and going to the refrigerator is physical activity; so is going for a walk. The amount of calories you use depends on your body weight and time. A person who weighs 200 pounds and walks for ten minutes uses more calories than a person who weighs 150 pounds and walks for ten minutes. All of your physical activities in a day use only about 25 percent of the total calories you consume. This means the physical activity from driving to the store, washing dishes, changing the channel on television … everything—only accounts for 25 percent of your total calories, and this even includes that 15 to 30 minutes of aerobic exercise three to five times a week.

So far, I've only accounted for 35 percent (10 digestion and 25 physical activity) of the calories you consume. What is the big user of calories? Pay attention, because here is one of the secrets to permanent weight loss and control.

Approximately 65 percent of the calories consumed in a day are used to supply the energy for the basic work of the body's cells to maintain life. This is energy used to keep the heart beating, the lungs breathing, all cells conducting activities, the nerves generating their continuous streams of electrical impulses. Basically, it's *all the functions that support life twenty-four hours a day even while you sleep.* This is called the *Basal Metabolic Rate* (BMR).

Your BMR can be measured in a laboratory when you are lying down and not digesting any food. By eliminating digestion and physical activity, electronic instruments can measure your calorie expenditure that is needed to support life. How can two people who are the same age, sex, height, and weight burn different amounts of calories if they are just lying down? How can Jane or Dick eat so much and stay thin?

The Secret to Permanent Weight Control

If you are accustomed to highlighting certain passages in a book with a yellow marker the way students do, then get ready to do that. How does a person obtain a high BMR? What's the secret? It's no secret to a nutritionist or dietitian. The key is the amount of *lean body tissue* or fat-free mass you have. Even when we sleep, lean tissue is more active metabolically than fat tissue. A person with lean tissue instead of fat tissue *burns more calories* and, therefore, gets to eat more calories. So Jane and Dick have more lean body tissue.

If you exercise and burn 200 calories every other day, the important point to remember is that you are keeping your muscles lean. Consequently, these muscles are using more calories the rest of the day, even at night.

It's the calorie demand of your BMR that keeps the fat people fat and the thin people thin.

Overweight people with lots of fat tissue will have a low calorie demand for their BMR. On the other hand, people with lean tissue will have a high calorie demand for their BMR. And as you now know, your *BMR accounts for 65 percent of your total calories.*

Oh, you can change. An overweight person can get thin, but it takes knowledge, commitment, and time. The longer one has been overweight, the longer it takes to become thin. But it is easy, once you have the know-how. You should not try to lose too much weight too fast.

Fasting and dieting lower your Basal Metabolic Rate, the opposite of what you want to do. Your body thinks there is a food shortage and it *slows down your BMR* so you can survive on fewer calories. Although you may lose a lot of weight, much of it will be muscle and not fat. If you decide to lose a lot of weight in a hurry, don't throw away your old clothes because the fat will be back. Ask Oprah Winfrey.

I mention Oprah Winfrey as an example, because she is nationally recognized and most people are familiar with her rapid weight loss. Many people have done exactly the same thing. Chances are, at her lowest weight, she was existing on very few calories. Who could stay on such a low calorie count? Why? Because when she lost a lot of weight in a short time, she lost muscle along with the fat and her BMR slowed down.

If you lose weight gradually (1/2 to 1 pound a week), you have these advantages:

1. Your body doesn't think there's a food shortage and your BMR doesn't slow down.
2. You lose fat and not muscle.

If you add moderate exercise the muscles become leaner, thereby raising their BMR. A higher BMR means you get to eat more.

I couldn't possibly go on without making a public apology to Oprah Winfrey. She is a person to be admired especially for her work on child abuse. I, in no way, meant to defame her. I mentioned her only because of the thousands of people who have done exactly the same thing. None of you should feel guilty. You were destined for failure before you started. Estimates are that 90 percent of the people who lose a lot of weight in a short time fail and go right back to their old weight or higher. Some people even start to think they are supposed to be overweight; how absurd.

I wasn't supposed to be overweight. I couldn't lose weight because I didn't understand nutrition; it's as simple as that. I didn't have a psychological problem or a glandular problem as many people imagine they do.

I suggest if you are overweight, you ask yourself two questions:

1. Do no more than 20 to 30 percent of my calories come from fat?
2. Do I exercise the equivalent of a 30 minute walk three to five times a week?

The starting point for weight loss and control is a resounding "YES" to both these questions.

Please don't fall victim to the celebrity who ballyhoos some weight loss program or product. You're smart, give yourself credit. If it sounds dumb or too good to be true, then it is. I say, to the baseball manager and former mayor who lend their names to diet programs, I feel you are doing a real disservice to your fans.

The Secret to Permanent Weight Control

You should know enough by now to realize that when you lose weight it could have been:

       1. WATER

       2. MUSCLE or

       3. FAT

Only when you understand how to lose fat can you achieve *permanent weight control.*

Please remember this. Rapid weight loss gets rid of muscle. This lost muscle is no longer on your body to burn calories. If you don't stick to a low calorie consumption you gain the weight back as fat. One pound of fat uses fewer calories than one pound of muscle. But, the one pound of fat takes up more space on your body than one pound of muscle.

If you have trouble visualizing this remember the old riddle; which weighs more a pound of feathers or a pound of steel? You're right, they both weigh a pound. Now, which one takes up more space? The pound of feathers would be about the size of a bed pillow. The pound of steel would be about the size of a golf ball. Muscle is like the golf ball and fat is like the pillow. When you lose muscle and replace it with fat, it's like tying all those pillows to various parts of your body; and you end up with one of the funny shaped bodies. I know a man shaped like a pear because his lean mass was replaced by fat.

Do you have an unusual shape? Now you know why. Chances are you have dieted before. I bet you lost three, four, or even five pounds in one week. Does this sound familiar? You didn't do your body any favor; you lost muscle! Are you eating fewer calories now than the first time you dieted? Of course you are, you have less muscle.

So, if you follow the guidelines in this book:

       1. Your fat consumption will be 20 to 30 percent of total calories.

       2. The weight (FAT) will come off slowly—about one pound a week.

       3. You will be eating more.

       4. Muscle will be retained or increased.

Maintaining your ideal weight should be easy and fun. And you should take pride in the fact that you are knowledgeable about nutrition and your good health.

Questions you now can answer:

1. Calories are used in three ways, name them.

   _____

   _____

   _____

2. A secret to permanent weight loss and control
   is that approximately ____ percent of the
   _____ consumed in a day are used
   to supply the energy for basic _____ of
   the _____ cells to _____ life.

3. The process that uses the most calories is?
   _____ metabolic _____.

4. What is Basal Metabolic Rate? All the
   _____ that _____ life.

5. How do you increase your BMR? Increase the
   amount of _____ body _____.

6. Why? _____ tissue is more _____ metabolically.

7. A person with _____ tissue instead of fat
   _____ burns more _____ and therefore
   gets to _____ more _____.

8. What keeps the fat people fat and the thin people
   thin? The calorie demand of your _____

9. On a low calorie diet you will slow your _____.

10. On a low calorie diet much of the weight you lose
    will be _____.

Bonus Question:

   What percent of your calories are used for:

Digesting Food	_____ %
Physical Activity	_____ %
Basal Metabolic Rate	_____ %

**OUR HEALTH ALWAYS SEEMS
MUCH MORE VALUABLE
AFTER WE LOSE IT**

CHAPTER 17

Overweight or Overfat

Don't exercise to lose weight. You should realize that if you exercise you may lose weight, but then again, you may gain weight. Confused? So was I, until, I began to understand what is happening when we exercise. On one hand, we are using more calories, so we should lose weight. On the other hand, exercise builds muscle tissue and muscle weighs more than fat. Some people who have started an exercise program have gained weight but still they fit into smaller sized clothes.

I like to think that an ideal diet controls our weight and keeps our arteries clear and that exercise makes our hearts strong. But in reality, the role of diet and exercise overlap. You should understand the importance of exercise in keeping your weight under control.

Carrying around too much body fat is a nuisance. Yet excess body fat is a common phenomenon in modern-day living. Few of today's occupations require vigorous physical activity, and much of our leisure time is spent in sedentary pursuits.

Recent estimates indicate that 34 million adults are considered obese (20 percent above desirable weight). Furthermore, over the past 20 years increased body fat levels have been seen in children and youth. It is noteworthy to mention that after infancy and early childhood, the earlier one becomes obese, the greater is the likelihood of that person remaining obese.

Excess body fat has been linked to such health problems as coronary heart disease, high blood pressure, osteoporosis, diabetes, arthritis and certain forms of cancer. Some evidence now exists showing that obesity has a negative effect on both health and longevity.

Exercise is associated with the loss of body fat in both obese and normal weight people. A regular program of exercise is an important component of any plan to help individuals lose, gain, or maintain their ideal weight.

Overweight and overfat, however, do not always mean the same thing. Some people are quite muscular and weigh more than the average for their age and height. However, body composition, the amount of fat versus lean body mass (muscle, bone, organs, and tissue) is within a desirable range. This is true for many athletes. Still numerous others weigh an average amount yet carry around too much fat.

Who would call Arnold Schwarzenegger overfat? Arnold is 6'2" tall and weighs between 210 and 215 pounds. In fact, he weighed as much as 250 pounds as a competitive bodybuilder. Yet, the height/weight table in Appendix 1 lists 197 as the maximum ideal weight for a man his height. Obviously, Arnold illustrates that muscle weighs more than fat but you don't look overweight.

In our society, however, overweight often implies overfat because excess weight is commonly distributed as excess fat. The addition of exercise to a weight control program helps control both body weight and body fat levels.

A certain amount of body fat is necessary for everyone. Experts say that the ideal percent of body fat for women should be about 20 percent, with 15 percent for men. Women with more than 30 percent fat and men with more than 25 percent fat are considered obese.

National fat averages are: 26 percent for men and 32 percent for women. Based on this, as a nation, we are obese. I consider this both an insult and a disgrace. Don't you? Possibly the worst effect this extra fat has on our bodies is that it wears out the heart.

When I weighed 180 pounds, I was over 20 percent above my ideal weight of 145 pounds; therefore, I fit the definition of obese. Most people don't like to be called obese. They may say they are plump, stocky, or big boned, but not obese. I, of course, was stocky.

The exceptions to this definition are the athletes who are over the ideal weight but have a low body fat content. Male athletes average 6 to 12 percent fat. Female athletes average 12 to 18 percent.

How much of your weight is fat can be assessed by a variety of methods including underwater (hydrostatic) weighing, skinfold thickness measurements and circumference measurements. Each requires a specially trained person to administer the test and perform the correct calculations. From the numbers obtained, a body fat percentage is determined. Assessing body composition has an advantage over the standard height-weight tables because it can help distinguish between "overweight" and "overfat."

An easy self-test you can do while standing is to pinch the thickness of the fat folds at your waist and abdomen. If you can pinch an inch or more of fat (make sure no muscle is included), chances are you have too much body fat. Here's another self-test. Take off all your clothes and stand in front of a mirror. Stop reading and go do this right now. WELL! Be honest now. Did you look overweight or overfat?

People who exercise appropriately increase lean body mass while decreasing their overall fat level. Depending on the amount of fat loss, this can result in a loss of inches without a loss of weight, since muscle weighs more than fat. However, with the proper combination of diet and exercise, both body fat and overall weight can be reduced if that's your goal.

THINK

SELF-ESTEEM

CHAPTER 18

How to Obtain Results With Energy Balance

Losing weight, gaining weight, or maintaining your weight depends on the amount of calories you take in and use up during the day. This is otherwise referred to as *energy balance*. Learning how to balance energy intake (calories in food) with energy output (calories expended through physical activity) will help you to achieve your desired weight.

The concept of energy balance is relatively simple. If you eat more calories than your body needs to perform your day's activities, the extra calories are stored as fat. If you do not take in enough calories to meet your body's energy needs, your body will go to the stored fat or muscle tissue to make up the difference. Exercise helps ensure that stored fat, rather than muscle tissue, is used to meet your energy needs. If you eat just about the same amount of calories to meet your body's energy needs, your weight will stay the same.

On the average, a person consumes between 800,000 and 900,000 calories each year. An active person needs more calories than a sedentary person, as physically active people require energy above and beyond the day's basic needs. All too often, people who want to lose weight concentrate on counting calorie intake while neglecting calorie output. The most powerful formula is the combination of dietary modification with exercise. By increasing your daily physical activity and decreasing your caloric input, you can lose excess weight in the most efficient and healthful way.

Each pound of fat your body stores represents 3,500 calories of unused energy. In order to lose one pound of fat, you would have to create a calorie deficit of 3,500 calories by either taking in 3,500 less calories over a period of time than you need or doing 3,500 calories worth of exercise. It is recommended that no more than two pounds (7,000 calories) be lost per week for lasting weight loss. This is a maximum. A half to one pound would be better.

If one pound of fat represents 3,500 calories, how many calories does a pound of lean body mass (muscle) represent? Hold your socks—480! Surprised? So was I. While your body must expend 3,500 calories to burn off a pound of body fat, *only about 480 calories are needed to get rid of a pound of lean body mass.* You could really lose weight by losing lean body mass, and this is what some diets cause. But, you don't want to lose lean body mass.

How about the diet that claims you can lose 10 pounds in a month? Sound to good to be true? Are you going to lose fat, water, or muscle? If you lose fat it means 35,000 calories (3,500 x 10 pounds) in one month! That's 8,750 calories in a week (35,000 divided by 4)! Let me tell you that's a lot of exercise to make sure you are losing fat and retaining your muscle. If the diet means you are losing water or muscle it's not a very good program. When you lose weight always ask yourself, did I lose water, muscle, or fat? You want to lose fat.

Adding 15 minutes of moderate exercise, say walking one mile, to your daily schedule will use up 100 extra calories per day. (Your body uses approximately 100 calories of energy to walk one mile, depending on your body weight.) Maintaining this schedule would result in an extra 700 calories per week used up, or a loss of about 10 pounds in one year, assuming your food intake stays the same.

To look at energy balance another way, just one extra slice of bread or one extra soft drink a day—or any other food that contains approximately 100 calories—can add up to ten extra pounds in a year if the amount of physical activity you do does not increase.

How to Obtain Results With Energy Balance

If you already have a lean figure and want to keep it, you should exercise regularly and eat a balanced diet that provides enough calories to make up for the energy you expend. If you wish to gain weight, you should exercise regularly and increase the number of calories you consume until you reach your desired weight. Exercise will help ensure that the weight you gain will be lean muscle mass, not extra fat.

Questions you now can answer:
1. Comparing the calories you take in with the calories you use is referred to as _____ _____.
2. Each pound of fat represents about _____ calories.
3. Each pound of lean body mass (muscle) represents about _____ calories.

> STOMACHS SHOULDN'T
> BE
> WAIST BASKETS

CHAPTER 19

Everyday Things That Help You

One thing is certain. Most people do not get enough exercise in their ordinary routines. All of the advances of modern technology—from electric can openers to power steering—have made life easier, more comfortable, and much less physically demanding. Yet our bodies need activity, especially if they are carrying around too much fat. Satisfying this need requires a definite plan—and—a commitment.

There are two main ways to increase the number of calories you expend:

1. Start a *regular exercise* program if you do not have one already.
2. Increase the amount of physical activity in your *daily routine*.

The best way to control your weight is a combination of the above. The sum total of calories used over time will help regulate your weight as well as keep you physically fit.

Before looking at what kind of regular exercise program is best, let's look at how you can increase the amount of physical activity in your daily routine to supplement your exercise program.

Recreational Pursuits

Gardening on weekends, bowling in the office league, family outings, an evening of social dancing, and many other activities provide added exercise. They are fun and can be considered an extra bonus in your weight control campaign.

Add More "Action" to Your Day

Walk to the neighborhood grocery store instead of using the car. Park several blocks from the office and walk the rest of the way. Walk up the stairs instead of using the elevator; start with one flight of steps and gradually increase. When you go to the mall, don't drive around looking for a parking spot close to the entrance. Park at the far corner of the lot; this will give you a block to walk. Quit taking the easy way out!

Change Your Attitude Toward Physical Activity

Instead of considering a short walk or trip to the files an annoyance, look at it as an added fitness boost. Look for opportunities to use your body. Bend, stretch, reach, move, lift and carry. Time-saving devices and gadgets eliminate drudgery and are a bonus to mankind. When they are substitutes for physical activity, however, they can take their toll on your health, vigor, and fitness.

It All Adds Up

These little bits of action are cumulative in their effects. Alone, each does not burn a huge amount of calories. But when added together, they can result in a sizable amount of energy used over the course of the day. And they will help to improve your muscle tone and flexibility at the same time.

Questions you now can answer:
1. Two areas you can increase the calories you expend are:
    A. _____
    B. _____

CHAPTER 20

The Proven Way to Results

Although any kind of physical movement requires energy (calories), the type of exercise that uses the most energy is *"aerobic"* exercise. The term "aerobic" is derived from the Greek word meaning "with oxygen." Jogging, brisk walking, swimming, biking, cross-country skiing and aerobic dancing are some popular forms of aerobic exercise.

Aerobic exercises use the body's large muscle groups in continuous, *rhythmic, sustained movement* and require oxygen for the production of energy. When oxygen is combined with food (which can come from stored fat), energy is produced to power the body's muscles. The longer you move aerobically, the more energy needed and the more calories used. Regular aerobic exercise will improve your *cardiorespiratory endurance*, the ability of your heart, lungs, blood vessels and associated tissues to use oxygen to produce energy needed for activity. You'll build a healthier body while getting rid of excess body fat.

In addition to aerobic exercising, supplement your program with muscle strengthening and stretching exercises. The stronger your muscles are, the longer you will be able to continue your aerobic activity, and the less chance you'll have of sustaining an injury.

Here are some tips to get you started:
1. Check with your doctor first.
> Since you are probably carrying around some extra "baggage," it is wise to get your doctor's "OK" before embarking on an exercise program.
2. Choose activities that you think you'll enjoy.
> Most people will stick to their exercise program if they are having fun, even though they are working hard.
3. Set aside a regular exercise time.
> Whether this means joining an exercise class or getting up a little earlier every day, make time for this addition to your routine and don't let anything get in your way. Planning ahead will help you get around interruptions in your workout schedule.
4. Set short term goals.
> Don't expect to lose 20 pounds in two weeks. It's taken awhile for you to gain the weight; it will take time to lose it. Keep a daily record of your progress and tell your friends and family about your achievements.
5. Vary your exercise program.
> Change exercises or invite friends to join you to make your workouts more enjoyable. (If you are doing something like walking or jogging, you should both have the same target heart rates, or one person will be going too fast or too slow.) There is no "*best*" *exercise*—just the one that works best for you.

Experts recommend that you do some form of aerobic exercise at least *three times a week* for a minimum of 20 continuous minutes. Of course, if that is too much, start with a shorter time span and gradually build up to the minimum. Then gradually progress until you are able to work aerobically for 20-40 minutes. If you need to lose a significant amount of weight, you may want to do your aerobic workout five times a week.

It is important to exercise at an intensity vigorous enough to cause your *heart rate and breathing* to increase. How hard you should exercise depends to a certain degree on your age and can be calculated by measuring your heart rate in beats per minute.

The heart rate you should maintain is called your *target heart rate*, and there are several ways you can determine this figure. The simplest method is to subtract your age from 220 and then calculate 60 to 80 percent of that figure. Beginners should maintain the 60 percent level; as you advance you can work up to the 80 percent level. A target heart rate chart is given in Appendix-16. This is just a guide, however, and people with any medical limitations should discuss this formula with their physician.

You can do different types of aerobic activities. Walk one day, ride a bike the next. Make sure you choose an activity that can be done regularly, and one you enjoy. The important thing to remember is not to skip too many days between workouts or your fitness benefits will be lost. If you must skip a few days, gradually work back into your routine.

The benefits of exercise are many. Producing *physically fit bodies* and providing an outlet for fun and socialization are just a couple that come to mind. When added to a weight control program, these benefits take on increased significance.

We have already noted that proper exercise can *help control weight* by burning excess body fat. It also has two other body trimming advantages:

1) Exercise builds muscle tissue and muscle uses calories up at a faster rate than body fat uses calories.

2) Exercise helps reduce unwanted inches and a firm, lean body looks slimmer even if your weight remains the same.

Remember that fat does not "turn into" muscle, as is often believed. Fat and muscle are two entirely different substances, and one cannot become the other; however, muscle does burn calories at a faster rate than fat. This directly affects your body's metabolic rate or energy requirement. Your basal metabolic rate (BMR) is the amount of energy required to sustain one's body's functions at rest. People with high levels of muscle tend to have higher BMRs and use more calories in the resting stage than people with lower levels.

Some studies have shown that the *metabolic rate stays elevated* for some time after vigorous exercise, resulting in the use of even more calories throughout your day.

Exercise also affects appetite. A lean person in good shape may actually eat more following increased activity, but the regular exercise will burn up the extra calories consumed. On the other hand, vigorous exercise has been reported to suppress one's appetite. Therefore, physical activity can be used as a positive substitute for between meal snacking.

The psychological benefits of exercise are as important as the physical benefits. Exercise *decreases stress* and relieves tension that might otherwise lead to overeating. Exercise results in physical fitness which in turn builds self-confidence, enhanced self-image, and a positive outlook. When you start to feel good about yourself, you are more likely to want to make other positive changes in your lifestyle that will help keep your weight under control.

In addition, exercise can be fun, provide recreation, and offer opportunities for companionship. The exhilaration and emotional release of participating in sports or other activities are a boost to mental and physical health. Pent-up anxieties and frustrations seem to disappear when you're concentrating on returning a serve, sinking a putt, or walking that extra mile.

Hopefully, you are now convinced that in order to successfully manage your weight you must include exercise in your daily routine.

It won't be easy, especially at the start. But as you begin to feel better, look better, and enjoy a new zest for life, you will be rewarded many times over for your efforts.

Tips to Keep You Going:
1. Adopt a specific plan and write it down.
2. Keep setting realistic goals as you go along; remind yourself of them often.
3. Keep a log to record your progress and keep it up to date.
4. Include weight and/or the percent of body fat measures in your log. Extra pounds can easily creep back.
5. Upgrade your fitness program as you progress.
6. Enlist the support and company of your family and friends.
7. Share your successes with others.
8. Avoid injuries by pacing yourself and including a warmup and cooldown period as part of every workout.
9. Reward yourself periodically for a job well done!

Questions you now can answer:

1. The type of exercise that uses the most energy
is_____.

2. Name two aerobic exercises _____ _____

3. Aerobic exercises use the body's large muscle groups in
_____, _____,and

_____ _____.

4. Aerobic exercise will improve your

_____ _____

5. What is the best exercise? _____

_____

6. You should exercise at least _____ _____
_____ _____ for 20 minutes.

7. It is important to exercise at an intensity vigorous enough
to cause your _____ _____ and _____
to increase.

8. You should exercise at your _____ _____

_____.

9. The benefits of exercise are:

_____

_____

_____

YOU CAN'T GET ANYWHERE UNLESS YOU START

CHAPTER 21

The Slower, Surer Way to Fitness

Walking is easily the *most popular* form of exercise. Other activities generate more conversation and media coverage, but none of them approaches walking in number of participants. Approximately half of the 165 million American adults (18 years of age and older) claim they exercise regularly, and two of every three list walking as one of their activities. Nearly 36 million adults walk for exercise daily and another 16 million do so two or three times a week.

Walking is the only exercise in which the rate of participation does not decline in the middle and later years. In a recent national survey, the highest percentage of regular walkers (39.4%) for any group was found among men 65 years of age and older.

In some weight-loss and conditioning studies, walking actually has proven to be more effective than running and other more highly-touted activities. That's because it's virtually injury-free and has the lowest dropout rate of any form of exercise.

Unlike tennis, running, skiing, and other activities that have gained popularity recently, walking has been widely practiced as a recreational and fitness activity throughout recorded history. Classical and early English literature seems to have been written largely by men who were prodigious walkers.

Both Emerson and Thoreau helped carry on the tradition in America. Among American presidents, the most famous walkers included Jefferson, Lincoln, and Truman.

Today, walking is riding a wave of popularity that draws its strength from a rediscovery of walking's utility, pleasures, and health-giving qualities.

People walk for many reasons: for pleasure, to rid themselves of tensions, to find solitude, or to get from one place to another. Nearly everyone who walks regularly does so, at least in part, because of a conviction that it is good exercise.

Often dismissed in the past as being "too easy to be taken seriously," walking recently has gained new respect as a means of improving physical fitness. Studies show that, when done briskly on a regular schedule, it can improve the body's ability to consume oxygen during exertion, thereby lowering the resting heart rate, *reducing blood pressure*, and *increasing* the *efficiency* of the *heart* and *lungs*. It also helps burn excess calories.

Since obesity and high blood pressure are among the leading risk factors for heart attack and stroke, walking offers protection against two major killers.

Walking takes longer to achieve the same results than does running and other more strenuous activities, but the difference is not as great as many people believe. A major university recently measured energy expenditure by 24 healthy male students during walks, jogs, and runs of varying speeds. One of their findings: jogging a mile in 8 1/2 minutes burns only 26 calories more than walking a mile in 12 minutes.

A study published in January of 1992 in the Journal of the American Medical Association suggests that walking at a 20 minute mile pace (3 miles per hour) is as good as jogging or other vigorous activity at raising levels of high-density lipoprotein (HDL). Participants in the study were randomly split into four groups: one group did not exercise and three groups walked three miles a day five times a week for a minimum of six months. The first group strolled at three miles per hour (mph), a 20 minute mile. The second group walked a brisk four mph, 15 minute mile. The final group walked at the aerobic pace of five mph, 12 minute mile.

The study found that exercise even at low intensities can provide a reduction in the risk of coronary disease. All three groups increased their blood HDL levels, "good" cholesterol by at least six percent.

The percentage of body fat also declined among all the walkers. Some of the women didn't lose weight; they just became leaner. The aerobic walkers lost four percent of their body fat. But the brisk walkers lost five percent, and the strollers lost the most, six percent. While the aerobic walkers burned 53 percent more calories, the strollers lost more body fat. This surprised researchers, but they now think that slow walks over a long distance is better for burning fat.

Studies done over 40 years ago have shown the increased risk of coronary heart disease that accompanies the sedentary life-style. One such study involved bus drivers and fare collectors on British double-decker buses. The drivers just sit and steer, but the conductors continually walk the bus, going up and down the stairs collecting fares. Who do you think had fewer heart attacks, the sedentary drivers or the active conductors? Bingo! Now you're catching on. The study showed that the conductors were much less likely to have heart attacks than the drivers.

Another study involved postal workers. Who do you think had fewer heart attacks, the clerks in the post office or the mail carriers walking routes? Right again! The walkers were far better off than their co-workers in the office.

There is a similarity between the recent study of walkers and these two older studies. Neither the mail carriers nor the bus conductors were walking at an aerobic pace.

The conclusion is this: you don't have to walk at a rapid pace to benefit your heart. Some people never start a walking program because they don't think they will enjoy walking fast. Now you know three mph is fine. How fast is that? Go to any store that sells treadmills and walk on one at three mph. For me it's slow, but for my father, who's 84, two and a half mph would be fast enough. It really comes down to you and your heart rate. You may feel better walking at 50 percent of your maximum heart rate and that's fine—just do it! Remember who you're doing this for—you. Walking should be fun, so do it at a pace that's enjoyable. In time, you may get so pumped up when you walk you may want to go faster. This is how it is for me. It's like a health high.

Like other forms of exercise, walking appears to have a substantial psychological payoff. Beginning walkers almost invariably report that they feel better and sleep better, and that their mental outlook improves.

Walking also can exert a favorable influence on personal habits. For example, smokers who begin walking often cut down or quit. There are two reasons for this. First, it is difficult to exercise vigorously if you smoke. Second, better physical condition encourages a desire to improve other aspects of one's life.

WALKING ADVANTAGES

In addition to the qualities it has in common with other activities, walking has several unique *advantages*. Some of these are:

1. Almost everyone can do it.

   You don't have to take lessons to learn how to walk. Probably all you need to do to become a serious walker is step up your pace and distance and walk more often.

2. You can do it almost anywhere.

   All you have to do to find a place to walk is step outside your door. Almost any sidewalk, street, road, trail, park, field, or shopping mall will do. The variety of settings available is one of the things that makes walking such a practical and pleasurable activity.

3. You can do it almost anytime.

   You don't have to find a partner or get a team together to walk, so you can set your own schedule. Weather doesn't pose the same problems and uncertainties that it does in many sports. Walking is not a seasonal activity, and you can do it in extreme temperatures that would rule out other activities.

4. It doesn't cost anything.

   You don't have to pay fees or join a private club to become a walker.

The only equipment required is a sturdy, comfortable pair of shoes. Although shoes are your only expense, they are critical. If your feet hurt, you will not want to walk. As Abraham Lincoln said, "When my feet hurt, I can't think." The best way to take care of your feet is with a good pair of shoes.

SHOES

Shoes need to be comfortable, provide good support, and prevent blisters or calluses. Here are some suggestions to help you make your selection:

1. Whatever kind of shoe you select, it should have an arch support and should elevate the heel one-half to three-quarters of an inch above the sole of the foot.
2. Choose a shoe with uppers made of materials that "breathe," such as leather or nylon mesh.

What makes a walk a workout? It's largely a matter of pace and distance. You move out at a steady clip that is brisk enough to make your heart beat faster and cause you to breathe more deeply.

WALKING STYLE

Here are some tips to help you develop an efficient walking style:

1. Hold your head erect and keep your back straight and your abdomen flat. Toes should point straight ahead and arms should swing loosely at your sides. (To get more exercise for your arms try "Power Walking"—discussed in the Chapter, "Power Walking")
2. Land on the heel of the foot and roll forward to drive off the ball of the foot. Walking only on the ball of the foot, or in a flat-footed style, may cause fatigue and soreness.
3. Take long, easy strides, but don't strain for distance. When walking up or down hills, or at a very rapid pace, lean forward slightly.
4. Breathe deeply. Breathe in through your nose and exhale out your mouth.

Weather will dictate your attire. As a general rule, you will want to wear lighter clothing than temperatures seem to indicate. Walking generates lots of body heat.

In cold weather, it's better to wear several layers of light clothing rather than one or two heavy layers. The extra layers help trap heat, and they are easy to shed if you get too warm. A wool watch cap or ski cap also will help trap body heat and provide protection for the head in very cold temperatures.

Walking poses few health risks. If you are free of serious health problems, you can start walking with confidence. Walking is not as strenuous as running, bicycling, or swimming and consequently involves almost no risk to health. Of course this statement assumes that you will use good judgment and not try to exceed the limits of your physical condition. I always recommend you talk to your doctor before you start an exercise program, how else will you know if you are free of serious health problems.

Most physicians recommend annual physical examinations for persons over 40 years of age. You should consult your physician before beginning any kind of exercise program.

Questions you now can answer:
1. The most popular form of exercise is _____.
2. Walking can not only lower the resting heart rate, it can also _____ blood _____ and increase the efficiency of the _____ and _____.
3. Walking has these advantages:

_____

_____

_____

_____

> THE MOUTH IS BOTH THE
> EXECUTIONER
> AND THE DOCTOR
> OF THE BODY

CHAPTER 22

Stretches, Warmup and Cool Down

Walking is good exercise for the legs, heart, and lungs, but it is not a complete exercise program. Persons who limit themselves to walking tend to become stiff and inflexible, with short, tight muscles in the back and backs of the legs. They also may lack muscle tone and strength in the trunk and upper body. These conditions can lead to poor posture and chronic lower-back pain, a problem that partially cripples or disables thousands of middle-aged and older Americans.

Prior to starting to exercise make sure you do some stretches. You should stretch for about five to ten minutes. This is a very important part of your exercise program if you want to *avoid* an *injury*. You should hold each stretch position for about 10 seconds without bouncing the muscle.

The exercises that follow are designed to increase *flexibility* and *strength* and to serve as a "warmup" for walking. Always do the exercises before walking. Other stretching exercises are listed in Appendix 19, but these are basic. You can do different stretches each day; it's a good idea to do stretches every day, even when you don't do an aerobic exercise.

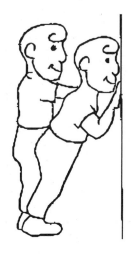

STRETCHER - Stand facing wall arms' length away. Lean forward and place palms of hands flat against wall, slightly below shoulder height, heels firmly on floor, and slowly bend elbows until forehead touches wall. Tuck hips toward wall and hold position for 20 seconds. Repeat exercise with knees slightly flexed. Do three to five times each way.

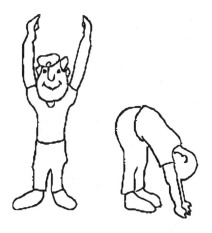

REACH and BEND - Stand erect with feet shoulder-width apart and arms extended over head. Reach as high as possible while keeping heels on floor and hold for 10 counts. Flex knees slightly and bend slowly at waist, touching floor between feet with fingers. Hold for 10 counts. (If you can't touch the floor, try to touch the tops of your shoes.) Repeat entire sequence 2 to 5 times.

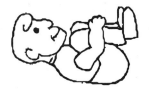

KNEE PULL - Lie flat on back with legs extended and arms at sides. Lock arms around legs just below knees and pull knees to chest, raising buttocks slightly off floor. Hold for 10 to 15 counts. (If you have knee problems, you may find it easier to lock arms behind knees.) Repeat exercise 3 to 5 times.

SITUP - Several versions of the situp are listed in reverse order of difficulty (easiest one listed first, most difficult one last). Start with the situp that you can do three times without undue strain. When you are able to do 10 repetitions of the exercise without great difficulty, move on to a more difficult version.

1. Lie flat on back with arms at sides, palms down, and knees slightly bent. Curl head forward until you can see past your feet, hold for three counts, then lower to start position. Repeat exercise 3 to 10 times.

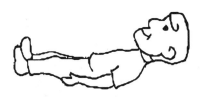

2. Lie flat on back with arms at sides, palms down, and knees slightly bent. Roll forward until upper body is at 45-degree angle to floor, then return to starting position. Repeat exercise 3 to 10 times.

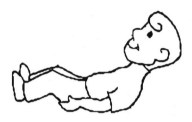

3. Lie flat on back with arms at sides, palms down, and knees slightly bent. Roll forward to sitting position, then return to starting position. Repeat exercise 3 to 10 times.

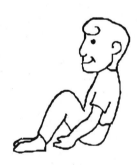

4. Lie flat on back with arms crossed on chest and knees slightly bent. Roll forward to sitting position, then return to starting position. Repeat exercise 3 to 10 times.

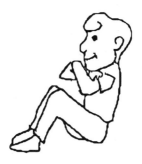

5. Lie flat on back with hands laced in back of head and knees slightly bent. Roll forward to sitting position, then return to starting position. Repeat exercise 3 to 15 times.

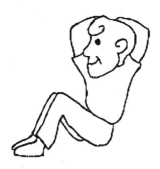

When you start to walk or ride the stationary bike or perform any other aerobic exercise, start out slowly. I walk at two miles per hour (mph) for five minutes to "warm up," and then I slowly increase my speed each minute until my heart rate hits my target. This takes five more minutes, and the treadmill is up to four and a half mph. I walk for 15 minutes with my heart rate at 130, and then I walk for five minutes at two mph to "cool down." The "*warm up*" and "*cool down*" are just as important as "*stretching*" to a complete exercise program. The cool down helps keep the blood from pooling below the waist. If you stop too fast, you may have insufficient circulation to the brain and heart.

When I ride the stationary bike, I pedal at 20 mph for five minutes for my "warm up." Then I pedal at 30 mph and slowly increase the tension as I monitor my heart rate till it reaches 130. I pedal for 15 minutes. Then I reduce the tension and slow down to 20 mph for five minutes as my "cool down." At the end of my cool down, my heart rate is just below 100.

Questions you now can answer:
1. Stretches are a very important part of an exercise program because they help avoid _____.
2. _____ exercises should be done before walking.
3. The _____ ____ and _____ _____ are just as important as _____ to a complete exercise program.

CHAPTER 23

Not Too Fast!

Now that you have decided to begin walking for exercise, you may be shocked at what poor shape you're in. If at first you have difficulty in meeting the standards suggested here, don't get discouraged. You can systematically build your stamina and strength to acceptable levels. Patience is the key to success. Some experts say that it takes a month of reconditioning to make up for each year of physical inactivity.

No one can tell you exactly how far or how fast to walk at the start, but you can determine the pace and distance by experimenting. I recommend that you begin by walking for 10 minutes at least four or five times a week at a pace that feels comfortable to you. (Remember to monitor your heart rate and not exceed 60 percent of maximum). If that proves to be too tiring or too easy, reduce or lengthen your time accordingly. I know many people who already walk 30 minutes a day at a slow pace. These people need to pay attention to their pulse and quicken their pace. Let your pulse be your guide.

Some elderly people and some people who are ill begin by walking for one or two minutes, resting a minute, and repeating this cycle until they begin to be fatigued. Where you have to start isn't important; it's where you're going that counts.

As your condition improves, you should gradually increase your time and pace. Your goal should be to walk at your target heart rate for 15 to 20 minutes. Even after you are in condition, you should start each walking session with *five minutes* of *easy walking* and end with *five minutes* of *easy walking*.

The *speed* at which you walk is *less important* than the *time* you devote to it. This time versus speed was discussed earlier, although I recommend that you walk as briskly as you feel comfortable. This will probably be between 50 and 80 percent of your maximum heart rate. I know this is a wide range, but this advice is aimed at a large audience. You may be between 20 and 90 years old, ideal weight or not, heart condition or not—the important point is to walk and be comfortable.

How fast should you walk? Besides feeling comfortable, the "*talk test*" can help you find the right pace. You should be able to carry on a conversation while walking. If you're too breathless to talk, you're going too fast. This advice goes for runners too.

The more often you walk, the faster you will improve. *Three workouts a week* are considered to be a "maintenance level" of exercise. More frequent workouts are required for swift improvement.

Listen to your body when you walk. If you develop dizziness, pain, nausea, or any other unusual symptom, slow down or stop. If the problem persists, see your physician before walking again.

Don't try to compete with others when walking. Even individuals of similar age and build vary widely in their capacity for exercise. Your objective should be to steadily improve your own performance, not to walk farther or faster than someone else.

The most important thing is simply to set aside part of each day for walking. No matter what your age or condition, it's a practice that can make you healthier and happier.

NOTE: You should consult with your doctor *before beginning an exercise program.*

Questions you now can answer:
1. Start each walk/run with five _____ of
   _____ walking and end with _____
   minutes of easy _____.
2. Speed is not as important as _____.
3. The _____ test can help you find the right speed.
4. You should at least have _____
   workouts a week.
5. You should consult with your doctor before beginning an
   _____ program.

LIFE IS HARD,

BY THE YARD;

BUT BY THE INCH,

LIFE'S A CINCH!

CHAPTER 24

Don't Exercise to Lose Weight

Why exercise? Ask this question and you get many answers—
to lose weight, to build muscles, to get in better shape. These
answers can be both right and wrong depending on whom you
ask. During my rehabilitation course, after my heart attack, it
was never taught that we were exercising to lose weight. Half
of the patients in the class did not need to lose weight.

So why exercise? If you ask bodybuilders, they will tell
you they are increasing the size of their muscles; in fact, they
will know what exercises are good for specific muscles.
During rehabilitation we were instructed not to be concerned
with the size of our muscles but with how efficient our
muscles were.

What about better shape? What do we mean by shape
anyway? Remember, I said earlier that half of my class did not
need to lose weight because they were already at their ideal
weight. Being in good shape means two things. The first is
not being overfat (not to be confused with overweight). The
second is to be cardiovascularly fit.

In class we were taught that we were exercising to improve
our *cardiovascular fitness*. What is cardiovascular fitness? To
keep it simple—it's the *heart*, *lungs*, and *muscles* being able to
process oxygen as *efficiently* as possible. In essence you get
the most benefit out of each pump of the heart. It makes the

heart stronger. This kind of fitness is what gives an athlete or you endurance.

In order to fully understand cardiovascular fitness, you need to understand the relationship between muscle, fat, and calories.

Think for a minute of a T-bone steak. See that fat around the outside and the fat running through the meat, we call marbling? Keep the idea of the T-bone steak in your mind as I talk about muscle and fat.

When I was younger, in my teens and twenties, I was in pretty good shape. My muscles did not have much marbling. They were "lean mass." As I got older and became less active, my muscles started to contain more fat as they marbled. As I continued to eat more calories than I burned, the excess was turned into fat and stored under the skin. This is *subcutaneous fat*, like the fat around that T-bone. This is the fat the doctors go after when they do a "fat suck" as I mentioned earlier. However, no doctor can get the fat out of your muscle (marbling)—only you can through exercise.

Bodybuilders and long distance runners have one thing in common. They both have muscles of lean mass with very little marbling. But, bodybuilders have done exercises to work on increasing the size of their muscles. If the bodybuilders are smart, they have included about 15 minutes a day of aerobic exercises such as jumping rope or riding a stationary bike in their routines. They know the heart is a muscle, and the way you exercise a muscle is to make it work. After all, they got their biceps bigger and stronger by working them. You work the heart by making it pump more than when it is just resting. The heart will respond to the exercise just like the biceps respond, it will get stronger. At rest, the heart beats about 72 beats per minute. During aerobic exercise, the goal is to increase the heart rate to between 60 and 80 percent of the maximum. (This is what's known as the "target heart rate" discussed earlier.)

Long distance runners are doing an aerobic exercise when they practice their sport. They are keeping their muscles lean and making their heart as strong as possible.

An aerobic exercise has other benefits. It makes the heart and all the muscles more efficient. It makes the heart stronger and increases the heart's pumping ability. It encourages *collateral circulation*, the growth of new smaller arteries, that can maintain blood flow around the heart when a major artery is blocked. I did not know this prior to my heart attack, but as you stimulate the heart through aerobic exercise, the heart will actually grow new arteries to supply the heart with blood. This benefit alone should encourage people to exercise.

A few years ago, a co-worker of mine found out during his flight medical that his EKG indicated he had suffered a major heart attack since his last EKG six months previously. He later needed a triple bypass. How could someone have a heart attack and not even know it? Collateral circulation! He appeared to be in great shape. He played tennis all the time, went on cross country bike rides, and was not overweight. He did say afterwards that he had had a mild chest discomfort on two occasions, once while playing tennis and once on a long bike ride. I never knew his cholesterol level.

This all happened prior to my heart attack, and I wasn't knowledgeable about cholesterol. It's interesting to note that because he was a pilot, he was required to have a resting EKG every six months. The collateral circulation probably saved his life at the time of the heart attack and the EKG probably saved him from a second and possibly fatal heart attack.

Of course, most people know the story of Jim Fixx, the best-selling author on exercise and running. He died, at the age of 52, of a heart attack while jogging. His total cholesterol at the time of death was 254.

These two stories further illustrate that exercise and the condition of your blood go hand in hand. Some people believe that if you exercise you don't need to be concerned with your cholesterol level. This is a misconception that could be fatal.

Some other benefits of an aerobic exercise program are:
1. It helps lower cholesterol and triglyceride levels in the blood.
2. It helps lower high blood pressure.
3. It helps maintain your ideal weight, and maintaining your ideal weight lessens your risk of heart attack, strokes, high blood pressure, some cancers, kidney diseases, diabetes, and a host of other illnesses.

Questions you now can answer:

1. You should exercise to improve your _____
   _____.

2. What is cardiovascular fitness? It's the _____
   lungs, and _____ being able to process _____
   as _____ as possible.

3. Fat stored under the skin is called _____
   _____

4. The growth of new smaller arteries around the heart is
   called _____   _____.

WHETHER YOU THINK
YOU CAN
OR THINK YOU CAN'T
YOU'RE RIGHT

CHAPTER 25

Why Thin People Stay Thin and Fat People Stay Fat

The resting heart rate starts to drop as you become fit. A resting heart rate in the low 50's is not uncommon for someone who is aerobically fit. By making the muscles more efficient—as the muscles lose their marbling and become lean mass—they alter their chemistry and increase their metabolic rate. Do you get that? As the muscles get rid of their marbling, they become more efficient at burning calories. This means that people with *lean muscle mass* tend to stay lean because their muscles are *efficient* at burning calories, and that fat people tend to stay fat because their muscles are *not* very *efficient* at *burning* calories. And the fatter they are the truer this becomes. It's a "Catch 22" since fit people get to eat more than fat people. Like to eat? Get fit! I'm sure that Arnold Schwarzenegger, at 210 pounds, gets to eat more than someone else who weighs the same but has more fat on their body.

Remember my earlier question about shape? Shape to me means two things: muscles that contain very little fat and a cardiovascular system that allows you to walk at a brisk pace while your heart rate stays within the target range.

I don't envy any overweight person. It's a long, hard process to get one's muscles back to lean mass where they can be more efficient at burning calories. It may take a year or more to reach your weight goal. You should aim to lose a half to one pound a week, no more than 52 pounds in a year. Your exercise goal should be 15 to 20 minutes at your target heart rate three to five times a week.

Remember, check with a doctor before you start any exercise program.

Questions you now can answer:
1. People with _____ _____ _____ tend to stay lean because their muscles are efficient at burning calories.
2. People tend to stay fat because their muscles are ____ very _____ at _____calories.

THE HUMAN BODY,
WITH PROPER CARE,
WILL LAST A
LIFETIME

CHAPTER 26

Power Walking

What do I do for exercise? I walk either on a treadmill or outside, and I ride an exercise bicycle. I alternate between walking and biking about five times a week thirty minutes each session. I have a pulse monitor that clips on my ear and gives me a reading of my pulse. I found the pulse monitor was well worth the investment. To me, this is easier than taking my pulse a few times each session.

I started doing something called power walking after I saw an article about it on television. I swing my arms when I walk, and I bend them at the elbow. My arms are straight on the back swing and as they come forward I bend them completely at the elbow. I have a one pound weight strapped around my wrists. Also, I open and close my hand, making a fist each time my arm swings. During the 30 minutes of exercising, I open and close my hand over 1,500 times. This is a great exercise for the fingers, hand, and forearm. Try it! While you're sitting there, open your hand; then make a fist and squeeze. I'll bet you can't do it 100 times without feeling tired. If exercising the fingers is protection against arthritis, this should be added to a walking routine. I do this same thing with my arms when I ride the exercise bike.

This additional use of your arms involves the upper body; this should satisfy those critics who say walking does not use the upper body.

How does power walking compare to jogging? I can only answer for me. By walking at four and a half to five mph I can achieve 80 percent of my maximum heart rate. Since I can meet my objective by walking, why should I jog and pound my knees? You may prefer jogging and that's OK; selecting an exercise is an individual thing.

> # HEALTH IS THE THING
> # THAT MAKES YOU FEEL
> # THAT <u>NOW</u> IS THE
> # BEST TIME OF THE YEAR

CHAPTER 27

What IS Your Exercise ?

What exercises should you do? You have many to choose from, so pick one you can have fun doing. Pick one that will raise your heart rate and keep it raised the whole time of the activity. If you have tried a particular exercise and quit, that does not mean there is not another one for you.

Give some long range thought to any exercise you try. If you are really into an exercise that is hard on your knees, you may find at age 40 or 50 that you have knee problems that are irreversible.

Walking
Of course, this is a good one. When you make it power walking, you include the upper body. It is not as traumatic to the knees and joints as running.

Running or Jogging
I tried this years before my heart attack. I found it hard to stay with although you may like it. Some drawbacks are: there are more injuries compared to walking; it is more traumatic to the knees and joints; it does not involve the upper body.

Cross Country Skiing
A great one whether done inside or out. It uses upper and lower body muscles and is not traumatic on your joints.

Swimming

Another good one because it is so easy on the joints. With a variety of strokes employed you get to use different muscles. This is my all-time favorite. The only drawback is pool availability. Call your local YMCA or parks department; they usually have time set aside for lap swimming. My mother-in-law, who's in her 70's and deathly afraid of water, took an aqua aerobic class at the "Y", partly because her doctor suggested it and partly to overcome her fear of water. What a great way to make new friends.

Bicycling

Whether done inside or outside, it is easy on your joints. If done outside, it is hard to keep a constant pulse, because of traffic, and it does not involve the upper body. It also can be a little dangerous. If done inside, a steady pace can be maintained and power riding can be added to use the upper body. Just swing those arms and flex those hands; add wrist weights if you like. I watch television; some people read a book. You can purchase a book holder that mounts to a stationary bike so that you can continue to use your upper body while you read.

Rowing Machine

Another good exercise. It exercises the lower and upper body muscles and is not traumatic on the joints.

Aerobic Dancing

This may be it for a lot of people. You may join a dance class just to see a routine or set one up in your home to your favorite music.

Step Climbing

This isn't my choice. Too much chance for a foot to slip resulting in a nasty ankle injury.

I'm sure you can think of many more exercises. Be sure to evaluate whether or not they are *aerobic*. Is your heart rate increased and steady? You should feel *comfortable*. If you feel uncomfortable or tired when your heart rate goes above 100, then don't. In time as you get into better shape, you will slowly be able to increase your speed and stay in a comfortable zone. Are you using your *legs, arms, back*, and *abdomen*? If not, you may need to add another routine. Is the activity *stressful to part of the body*?

These exercises can be called "*endurance exercises*" because they increase a person's endurance. Professional athletes (like marathoners, bicyclists, and cross-country skiers) who compete in endurance sports end up having larger hearts than nonathletes. Studies at the National Heart Institute in Bethesda proved that the "endurance hearts" of long distance runners are bigger. With endurance training, the heart grows larger and its filling capacity is increased. In a trained athlete the volume of the heart at rest may be twice that of the nonathlete. This may be reflected in a resting pulse as low as 28 beats per minute, and a low blood pressure reading.

This is not to say that if you exercise 30 minutes a day, your heart will double its output. But don't be surprised if your endurance for all activity goes up and your resting pulse goes down. Your blood pressure may also go down if it has been high. Not so long ago, if a nurse or doctor checked your pulse and it was in the 50's they would get concerned. Now, if they know you're in an aerobic exercise program, they consider a low pulse normal.

If you choose an activity that requires the purchase of equipment, you have two things to consider. Make sure you like the activity before you purchase the equipment. You may want to join an exercise club or YMCA at least on a short trial offer to evaluate what equipment you like. Give each exercise machine a fair try. It took me a few times on a treadmill to be able to walk without holding on to the side rail. The second thing is, buy something made well. I have had a Schwinn stationary bicycle for ten, trouble free years. I can say the same for my treadmill, a Pace Master built by Aerobics Inc.

Some considerations of a well-built treadmill are: the horsepower of the motor, the size of the walking surface, the elevation capabilities, the range of speed, and naturally, the guarantee features.

One thing most people don't consider when they pick an activity is what will they be thinking about when they do the activity. This is more important than you realize. Some activities require your utmost concentration, thereby taking your mind off the stresses of the day. A friend of mine plays handball because his mind is so involved with the activity he forgets all about work and other problems. Other activities are done so effortlessly your mind is free.

Oliver Wendell Holms wrote, "In walking, the will and the muscles are so accustomed to working together and perform their task with so little expenditure of force that the intellect is left comparatively free." I found this to be true for me. While walking outside I have solved problems and come up with many ideas. While on the stationary bike or treadmill, my mind has been free to watch television or listen to music. Yet, when I swim, all my concentration is on swimming.

Remember, the right exercise is the one that's enjoyable for you. You may have to try a few before you find one you like.

Questions you now can answer:
1. Things to consider when you evaluate an exercise:
   A. _____ - is your heart rate increased and steady?
   B. Is it _____?
   C. Are you using _____ ?
   D. Is the activity _____ ?
   _____ ?
2. Aerobic exercises are also _____ exercises.

DESTINY SHAPES THE FUTURE,
BUT
FAT INTAKE SHAPES OUR
ENDS AND OUR MIDDLE

CHAPTER 28

Putting What You Know to Work

By now you should know quite a bit about nutrition and exercise. The more you know, the easier it is to lose weight or lower cholesterol. So how do you put this knowledge to work? That depends on if you are five pounds overweight or one hundred or more pounds overweight. It also depends on whether you have an ideal blood cholesterol level or a reading that is extremely high. In other words, each program should be individualized to fit a person.

The first step is to write down some information about yourself so that you know where you are now. Then you can track your improvement. Fill in the health information page in this chapter. You need your weight, blood pressure, pulse; and then from a blood test, you'll find the total cholesterol, HDL, LDL, and triglycerides.

If you are much overweight, don't be surprised if you also have high cholesterol and high blood pressure. And the more overweight you are, the more likely this will be true. Many people find that when they reach their ideal weight they no longer have high blood pressure or high cholesterol.

The very least you should do is have a working knowledge of the food you eat—I mean the amount of cholesterol in a food and the percent of calories that come from fat.

To do this, make lists of foods you eat for breakfast, lunch, and supper and show the calories, cholesterol, and fat in each. I provided a partial list in the next chapter. Of course, everyone's lists will be different.

The main reason for making your lists is for you to become aware of cholesterol and fat in various foods you eat. Making the lists will be easy. With the appendices and the "Percent of Calories From Fat Chart" (see Appendix 17), your job is simple.

With each passing day you will find you are adding fewer and fewer items to your lists. At the end of thirty days, your lists will be almost complete and you will add something very infrequently. By seeing the amount of cholesterol and fat you consume, you will be more likely to substitute foods that are low in fat for some you eat that are high in fat. Since the foods you substitute are on your lists, you must like them. Therefore, you will still be eating things you like but ones which are better for you. No one should eat things they don't like.

Don't say, "This is too hard, I can't write it down." If you've ever tried any diet program, you have already put out more physical and mental effort than is required here. Making your lists is a mental effort. Eating a good item on your list instead of a bad item is a physical effort. Many other programs require that you eat or drink their items. This is a difficult physical effort that is hard to stick to.

This program's premise is that anything is easy if you have know-how. You need to be informed to be successful. Your goal should be to eat nothing unless you know the amount of fat and cholesterol in it. Do it for one month. What have you got to lose—fat and cholesterol?

Making lists and some informed substitutions may be all you need to do. This might be called the first level of knowledge.

The second level would be to write down what you eat each day for 30 days making changes where necessary to eat nutritiously. This only takes 15 minutes a day. I did it watching television at the end of the day. It didn't cost me any time as I did it during commercials.

To help you do this, I have included some charts. One chart you saw earlier is the "Percent of Calories From Fat Chart." For many items without labels I have included an appendix, which lists various foods and shows cholesterol, fat, and the percent of calories from fat.

The next chart shows the recommended amount of fat, protein, and carbohydrates a person should get for his/her total calories in a day. If, for example, you decide you should have 1,600 calories a day in order to lose one pound a week, then find 1,600 calories under the column labeled total calories. Next go across to the right and under the column labeled fat you will see calories (480) and grams of fat (53) that represents 30 percent of the total calories. Find the calories and grams of fat that are right for you. Do not exceed the grams of fat each day.

CALORIES AND RECOMMENDED PERCENT CHART

TOTAL CALORIES	FAT 30 % grams	CARBOHYDRATE 58 % grams	PROTEIN 12 % grams
1,000	300 K	580 K	120 K
	33 g	145 g	30 g
1,200	360	696	144
	40	174	36
1,400	420	812	168
	46	203	42
1,600	480 K	928	192
	53 g	232	48
1,800	540	1044	216
	60	261	54
2,000	600	1160	240
	66	290	60
2,200	660	1276	264
	73	319	66
2,400	720	1392	288
	80	348	72
2,600	780	1508	312
	86	377	78
2,800	840	1624	336
	93	406	84
3,000	900	1740	360
	100	435	90
100	30	58	12
	3	14	3

K = calories   g = grams
NOTE: Fat can be reduced to 20 percent with carbohydrates making up the difference.

Health Information

Date _____ Height _____ Weight _____

Ideal Weight _____

Pulse _____ Blood Pressure _____

Cholesterol _____ HDL _____ LDL _____

Triglycerides _____

Age _____ Target Heart Rate _____

You should weigh in once a week at the same time of day, preferably in the morning when you wake up. As discussed already, the other items vary as to how often you need to have them checked, but when you do, write them down.

THE DICTIONARY

IS THE ONLY PLACE

SUCCESS

COMES BEFORE

WORK

CHAPTER 29

37 Days to Results You Will Love

In this chapter you will find a daily log for 30 days. Write down your calorie and fat grams allowed each day. You may want to cut back to 20 percent on the fat. There is also a place to keep track of cholesterol and exercise. How much of the log you use is up to you. If you don't write down what you eat each day, at least try it once a week to see what your daily percent of calories from fat is on a typical day.

After 30 days you may have changed your habits enough that you won't need the log. It surely shouldn't take more than 90 days. But I would continue with the breakfast, lunch, and supper lists, adding to them as you try new items. In this way you will stay aware of how much fat and cholesterol are in the foods you eat. Continue to weigh-in once a week with a goal of half to one pound loss per week if you want to lose weight. If you cut a lot of fat from your meals, you may find you are losing more than one pound a week. Increase your carbohydrates and check your protein. You do not want to lose more than one pound a week.

37 DAY CHECKLIST

First seven days

1. No eating or exercise changes to your normal routine.
2. Fill in the health information in the previous chapter.
3. Call some local hospitals or the American Heart Association to find out where you can get a cholesterol blood test.
4. Reread chapters that apply to you and answer all questions.
5. Start making your lists for breakfast, lunch, and supper. Use the format in this chapter. Use the percent of fat chart.
6. Give some serious thought to an exercise program that fits your age and current condition. Consult with your doctor.
7. Decide whether you want to keep track of calories each day, grams of fat, or just make a few substitutions.
8. On day seven make out a supper menu for the next seven days.
9. On day eight start your program. Fill out a daily log even if you elected to keep track of very little information.
10. Continue to update your food lists. Your breakfast list will be 90 percent done.
11. If you had your blood tested at a screening where your doctor may not get the results and your cholesterol was over 200, make sure your doctor is made aware of the reading.
12. Weigh in once a week. If you lose over one pound add some carbohydrates.
13. By the end of 37 days you should be able to sit down to any meal and have a good idea what percent of calories come from fat.

Breakfast - Lunch - Supper

When I first decided to write down everything I ate, I thought it would be a difficult job. But I was wrong. I started by making a master list for Breakfast, Lunch, and Supper. Within a month, most things I ate were on the lists. During the day I would jot down each item I ate. Then each night it took me only about ten minutes to get my calorie and cholesterol count total for the day. Once in a while I would try something new and add it to the master lists. If it is a recipe, add all the ingredients and divide by the number of servings. If it's not on the lists, get the information off the label or from the appendices and add it to the lists. In a short time these lists will reflect the foods you normally eat. Extra meal list pages can be found in this chapter.

The lists show:
1. CAL = Calories
2. CHOL = Cholesterol
3. FAT = Grams of Fat
4. % FAT = Percent of Calories from Fat

Symbols are:
1. S = serving
2. T = Tablespoon
3. t = teaspoon
4. tr = Trace
5. C = Cup
6. oz = Ounce
7. < = less than
8. sl = slice

A HEART ATTACK CAN SAVE YOUR LIFE

BREAKFAST	AMOUNT	CAL	CHOL	FAT	% FAT
Cereal - Cheerios	1 S	110	0	1	8
Cereal - Chex - wheat	1 S	110	0	0	0
Cereal - Grape Nuts	1 S	110	0	0	0
Cereal - Just Right	1 S	100	0	0	0
Cereal - Just Right with fruit	1 S	140	0	1	6
Cereal - Oat Bran	1 S	120	0	2	15
Cereal - Oat Meal	1 S	110	0	2	16
Cereal - Quaker 100% Natural (good snack)	1 S	110	0	2	16
Cereal - Shredded Wheat	1 S	110	0	0	0
Cereal - Total Raisin Bran	1 S	130	0	1	7
Coffee	1 C	0	0	0	0
Egg Beaters	2	50	0	0	0
Fruit - see dessert list					
Jelly - Grape	2 t	35	0	0	0
Juice - Orange	1 C	110	0	tr	tr
Margarine	1 T	100	0	11	99
Milk - Whole	1 C	150	34	8	48
Milk - 2 percent	1 C	120	22	5	37
Milk - Nonfat	1 C	85	4	tr	tr
Sugar	1 t	15	0	0	0
Syrup	1 T	160	0	0	0
Syrup - lite	1 T	80	0	0	0
Pancakes - Aunt Jemima	1 S	210	0	0	0

(made with Eggbeaters, non-fat milk, no oil, and non-stick pan) Buy a brand with zero fat and leave out the oil when mixing.

List YOUR foods here.

BREAKFAST	AMOUNT	CAL	CHOL	FAT	% FAT
_____	___	___	___	___	___
_____	___	___	___	___	___
_____	___	___	___	___	___
_____	___	___	___	___	___
_____	___	___	___	___	___
_____	___	___	___	___	___
_____	___	___	___	___	___

BREAKFAST	AMOUNT	CAL	CHOL	FAT	% FAT
_____	____	___	___	___	___
_____	____	___	___	___	___
_____	____	___	___	___	___
_____	____	___	___	___	___
_____	____	___	___	___	___
_____	____	___	___	___	___
_____	____	___	___	___	___
_____	____	___	___	___	___
_____	____	___	___	___	___
_____	____	___	___	___	___
_____	____	___	___	___	___
_____	____	___	___	___	___
_____	____	___	___	___	___
_____	____	___	___	___	___
_____	____	___	___	___	___
_____	____	___	___	___	___
_____	____	___	___	___	___
_____	____	___	___	___	___
_____	____	___	___	___	___
_____	____	___	___	___	___
_____	____	___	___	___	___
_____	____	___	___	___	___
_____	____	___	___	___	___
_____	____	___	___	___	___
_____	____	___	___	___	___
_____	____	___	___	___	___
_____	____	___	___	___	___
_____	____	___	___	___	___
_____	____	___	___	___	___
_____	____	___	___	___	___
_____	____	___	___	___	___
_____	____	___	___	___	___
_____	____	___	___	___	___
_____	____	___	___	___	___

A HEART ATTACK CAN SAVE YOUR LIFE

LUNCH	AMOUNT	CAL	CHOL	FAT	% FAT
Bread - Bagel 1		150	0	1	6
Bread - Pita.................... 1		165	0	1	5
Bread - Wheat...............1 S		65	0	1	13
Bread - White ....1 S		65	0	1	13
Cheese - American - Cheddar ....1 oz.		110	28	9	73
Cheese - Weight Watchers...........1 S		50	10	2	35
Cheese - Cream...........1 oz.		100	32	10	90
Cheese - Kraft Philadelphia - FREE....1 oz.		25	5	0	0
Crackers - Nabisco Graham....................... 2		60	0	1	15
Crackers - Saltine............. 4		50	0	1	18
Crackers - Nabisco Fat Free 5		50	0	0	0
Dressing - French ....1 T		101	3	6	53
Dress. French - lite.........1 T		30	0	1	30
Dress. Thousand Is. ....1 T		112	tr	8	64
Dress. Thous. Is./lite ......1 T		61	tr	2	29
Dress. S & W oil free White wine & Vinegar....1 T		16	0	0	0
Meat - See Supper list					
Miracle Whip - Free........1 T		20	0	0	0

List YOUR foods here.

LUNCH	AMOUNT	CAL	CHOL	FAT	% FAT

LUNCH	AMOUNT	CAL	CHOL	FAT	% FAT

SUPPER	AMOUNT	CAL	CHOL	FAT	% FAT
Applesauce	1 C	105	0	tr	tr
Beans - Van Camps	8 oz.	220	0	2	8
Fries - Oreida (lite)	3 oz.	100	0	3	27
Healthy Choice - frozen dinner					
Pasta Shells Marinara	1	360	25	3	7
Sweet & Sour Chicken	1	310	50	5	14
MEAT					
Bacon - Canadian	2 sl.	85	27	4	42
Bacon - Regular	3 sl.	110	16	9	73
Steak - Sirloin	3 oz.	240	77	15	56
Chicken - light meat	3.5 oz	153	75	4	23
Ham - steak	3.5 oz	122	45	4	31
Beef, top round					
Lean	3.5 oz	191	84	6	29
Haddock	3.5 oz	112	74	1	7
Halibut	3.5 oz	140	41	3	19
Tuna	3.5 oz	184	49	6	31

For more Meats see Appendices 2, 3, and 4.

Pizza - cheese 15"					
diameter	1/8	290	56	9	28
Potato	1	220	0	tr	tr
Rice	1 C	225	0	tr	tr
Sour Cream - Fat Free	2 T	18	0	0	0
Spaghetti sauce	1 C	25	0	0	0
Spaghetti pasta	1 C	210	0	1	4

Vegetables - Most vegetables have about 25 calories per serving with no cholesterol and only a trace of fat. See Appendix 14.

List YOUR foods here.

SUPPER	AMOUNT	CAL	CHOL	FAT	% FAT
_____	___	__	__	__	__
_____	___	__	__	__	__
_____	___	__	__	__	__
_____	___	__	__	__	__
_____	___	__	__	__	__
_____	___	__	__	__	__
_____	___	__	__	__	__
_____	___	__	__	__	__
_____	___	__	__	__	__

SUPPER	AMOUNT	CAL	CHOL	FAT	% FAT
_____	_____	____	____	___	_____
_____	_____	____	____	___	_____
_____	_____	____	____	___	_____
_____	_____	____	____	___	_____
_____	_____	____	____	___	_____
_____	_____	____	____	___	_____
_____	_____	____	____	___	_____
_____	_____	____	____	___	_____
_____	_____	____	____	___	_____
_____	_____	____	____	___	_____
_____	_____	____	____	___	_____
_____	_____	____	____	___	_____
_____	_____	____	____	___	_____
_____	_____	____	____	___	_____
_____	_____	____	____	___	_____
_____	_____	____	____	___	_____
_____	_____	____	____	___	_____
_____	_____	____	____	___	_____
_____	_____	____	____	___	_____
_____	_____	____	____	___	_____
_____	_____	____	____	___	_____
_____	_____	____	____	___	_____
_____	_____	____	____	___	_____
_____	_____	____	____	___	_____
_____	_____	____	____	___	_____
_____	_____	____	____	___	_____
_____	_____	____	____	___	_____
_____	_____	____	____	___	_____
_____	_____	____	____	___	_____
_____	_____	____	____	___	_____
_____	_____	____	____	___	_____
_____	_____	____	____	___	_____
_____	_____	____	____	___	_____
_____	_____	____	____	___	_____
_____	_____	____	____	___	_____
_____	_____	____	____	___	_____

DESSERTS & MISC.	AMOUNT	CAL	CHOL	FAT	% FAT
Angel food cake	1 S	125	0	tr	tr
Beer	1	150	0	0	0
Chocolate	1 oz	160	10	9	50
Cookies - Nabisco Fat Free Fig Bars	1	70	0	0	0
Cookies - Nabisco Cranberry Newtons	1	70	0	0	0
Cookies - Nabisco Ginger snaps	2	60	0	1	15
Cracker Jack	1 oz	120	0	3	22
Fruit Bar	1	45	0	0	0

Fruit - Most Fruits have about 40 calories per serving with no cholesterol and only a trace of fat. See Appendix 14.

	AMOUNT	CAL	CHOL	FAT	% FAT
Ice Cream	1 C	269	59	14	48
Ice Cream - lite	1 C	90	5	3	30
Popcorn - lite	3 C	70	0	3	27
Pretzel	1 oz	110	0	0	0
Pudding (nonfat milk)	1/2 C	136	2	tr	tr
Sherbet, orange	1 C	270	14	4	13
Soda - most	12 oz	150	0	0	0
Tapioca - Nonfat milk & Egg beaters	1 S	85	2	tr	tr

Also see Appendix 6.
List YOUR foods here.

DESSERTS & MISC.	AMOUNT	CAL	CHOL	FAT	% FAT
_____	__	__	__	__	__
_____	__	__	__	__	__
_____	__	__	__	__	__
_____	__	__	__	__	__
_____	__	__	__	__	__
_____	__	__	__	__	__
_____	__	__	__	__	__
_____	__	__	__	__	__
_____	__	__	__	__	__
_____	__	__	__	__	__
_____	__	__	__	__	__
_____	__	__	__	__	__

DESSERTS & MISC.	AMOUNT	CAL	CHOL	FAT	% FAT
——————	——	——	——	——	——
——————	——	——	——	——	——
——————	——	——	——	——	——
——————	——	——	——	——	——
——————	——	——	——	——	——
——————	——	——	——	——	——
——————	——	——	——	——	——
——————	——	——	——	——	——
——————	——	——	——	——	——
——————	——	——	——	——	——
——————	——	——	——	——	——
——————	——	——	——	——	——
——————	——	——	——	——	——
——————	——	——	——	——	——
——————	——	——	——	——	——
——————	——	——	——	——	——
——————	——	——	——	——	——
——————	——	——	——	——	——
——————	——	——	——	——	——
——————	——	——	——	——	——
——————	——	——	——	——	——
——————	——	——	——	——	——
——————	——	——	——	——	——
——————	——	——	——	——	——
——————	——	——	——	——	——
——————	——	——	——	——	——
——————	——	——	——	——	——
——————	——	——	——	——	——
——————	——	——	——	——	——
——————	——	——	——	——	——
——————	——	——	——	——	——

149

A HEART ATTACK CAN SAVE YOUR LIFE

FAST FOODS	AMOUNT	CAL	CHOL	FAT	% FAT
McDONALD'S					
Hamburger.................... 1		255	37	9	31
Cheeseburger 1		305	50	13	38
Chunky Chicken					
Salad......................... 1		150	78	4	24
French Fries - small.......... 1		220	0	12	49
French Fries large 1		400	0	22	49
Hotcakes w/margarine					
& syrup (2 pats)............ 1		440	8	12	24
McLean Deluxe 1		302	60	10	28
McLean Deluxe					
w/Cheese................... 1		370	75	14	34
Milk Shake - Vanilla 1		290	10	1.3	4
Milk Shake - Chocolate...... 1		320	10	1.7	5
Muffin - Fat free					
Apple Bran Muffin.......... 1		180	0	0	0
Sausage McMuffin					
w/Egg........................ 1		430	270	25	52
KENTUCKY FRIED CHICKEN					
Original Recipe .... 2 pieces		393	164	26	59
Extra Crispy........... 2 pieces		544	168	37	61
LONG JOHN SILVERS					
Baked - 3 piece fish					
Lemon Crumb............... 1		150	110	1	6
Batter Fried Fish.............. 1		210	30	12	51
3 Pc. Fish Dinner............. 1		780	75	34	39
3 Pc. Chicken					
Planks Dinner............... 1		860	160	37	38
Ocean Chef Salad............. 1		150	40	5	30
without dressing					

FAST FOODS	AMOUNT	CAL	CHOL	FAT	% FAT
BURGER KING					
Chicken Sandwich .... 1 BK Broiler		267	45	8	27
Chunky Chicken Salad 1		142	49	4	25
Double Cheeseburger........ 1		483	100	27	50
Double Whopper 1		844	170	53	56
French Fries - med. 1		372	0	20	48
Ocean Catch - Fish........... 1 Filet Sandwich		479	45	33	62
Vanilla Shake 1		334	33	10	26
Whopper..................... 1		614	91	36	52

You can ask any fast food restaurant manager if he/she has a booklet containing nutrition information. You can write to the below addresses for their booklet:

 Burger King Corporation
 17777 Old Cutler Road
 Miami, Fl. 33157
 Telephone 1-800-"YES"-1-800
 Kentucky Fried Chicken
 P.O. Box 32070
 Louisville, Ky. 40232
 Long John Silvers, Inc.
 101 Jerrico Drive
 P.O. Box 11988
 Lexington, Ky. 40579
 Telephone 1-800-342-3669
 McDonald's Nutrition Information Center
 McDonald's Plaza
 Oak Brook, Illinois, 60521

You should check the current fast food items as changes are being made to satisfy health conscious consumers. McDonalds appears to be the leader in this area.

DAILY LOG   DATE _____/_____/_____
ALLOWED--Calories _____ Fat (g) _____ 20 percent
Cholesterol _____ _____ Fat (g) _____ 30 percent

Breakfast	Calories	CHOL.	Fat (g)
_____	_____	_____	_____
_____	_____	_____	_____
_____	_____	_____	_____
_____	_____	_____	_____
_____	_____	_____	_____
_____	_____	_____	_____
Lunch			
_____	_____	_____	_____
_____	_____	_____	_____
_____	_____	_____	_____
_____	_____	_____	_____
_____	_____	_____	_____
_____	_____	_____	_____
Supper			
_____	_____	_____	_____
_____	_____	_____	_____
_____	_____	_____	_____
_____	_____	_____	_____
_____	_____	_____	_____
_____	_____	_____	_____
TOTAL	_____	_____	_____

Percent calories from fat--9 X (_____) total fat grams equals calories from fat (_____) divided by (_____) total calories = _____ percent calories from fat.
Exercise: type _____   time _____
Glasses of water: (8) _____ This amount of water may be too much for some individuals, ask your doctor.
NOTE: You will find additional logs at the end of the book. The following seven days worth of meals are for 1,500 calories. You may need to adjust your calories above or below that figure. Notice how easy it was to keep the percent of calories from fat below 30 percent. You will get lots to eat if you keep the fat below 30 percent. The more fat you cut out the more you will get to eat. I included margarine a few times; the more you can cut back on this high fat item the better off you will be.
NOTE: Meat and Poultry items are 3.5 oz. cooked unless otherwise stated.

DAILY LOG   DATE _____ / _____ / _____   DAY 1
ALLOWED--Calories   <u>1500</u>   Fat (g) <u>33</u>   20 percent
Cholesterol <u>150</u>   Fat (g) <u>50</u>   30 percent

Breakfast	Calories	CHOL.	Fat (g)
Coffee & sugar	15	0	0
Orange Juice 1/2 C	50	0	0
Oat Bran	120	0	2
Milk (nonfat) 1C	80	5	0
Any Fruit	40	0	0
Lunch			
Bread 2 slices	140	0	2
Tomato	30	0	0
Miracle Whip Free	20	0	0
Ham 3 slices	60	30	1
Any Fruit	40	0	0
Applesauce	40	0	0
Fig Newton - 2	140	0	0
Milk	80	5	0
Supper			
Chicken 3 oz.	160	75	4
Rice 1/3 C	80	0	0
Carrots	25	0	0
String Beans	25	0	0
Soda	150	0	0
Roll	100	0	1
Margarine - 1 T	<u>100</u>	<u>0</u>	<u>11</u>
TOTALS	1495	115	21

Percent calories from fat--9 X 21= 189 calories from fat
divided by 1495 total calories = 13 percent calories from fat.
Exercise: type _____   time _____
Glasses of water: (8) _____

DAILY LOG   DATE ____/____/____   DAY 2
ALLOWED--Calories   1500   Fat (g) 33   20 percent
Cholesterol 150   Fat (g) 50   30 percent

Breakfast	Calories	CHOL.	Fat (g)
Coffee & sugar	15	0	0
Total Rasin Bran	130	0	1
Bread 2 slices	140	0	2
Milk (nonfat) 1C	80	5	0
Any Fruit	40	0	0
Jelly - 4 t	70	0	0
Lunch			
Bread 2 slices	140	0	2
Tomato	30	0	0
Miracle Whip Free	20	0	0
Tuna 2 oz.	110	30	1
Any Fruit	40	0	0
Baked Beans	110	0	1
Supper			
Veal Cutlet	156	128	2
Two Veg.	50	0	0
Milk	80	5	0
Fruit	40	0	0
Roll	100	0	1
Margarine 1 T	100	0	11
Popcorn 3 C	100	0	3
TOTALS	1551	168	24

Percent calories from fat--9 X 24 = 216 calories from fat divided by 1551 total calories = 14 percent calories from fat.
Exercise: type _____   time _____
Glasses of water: (8) _____

DAILY LOG   DATE ____/____/____   DAY 3
ALLOWED--Calories <u>1500</u>   Fat (g) <u>33</u>   20 percent
Cholesterol <u>150</u>   Fat (g) <u>50</u>   30 percent

Breakfast	Calories	CHOL.	Fat (g)
Coffee & sugar	15	0	0
Post Grape Nuts	110	0	0
English Muffin	140	0	1
Milk (nonfat) 1C	80	5	0
Any Fruit	40	0	0
Jelly 2 T	120	0	0
Lunch			
Bread 2 slices	140	0	2
Cheese - Weight	----	---	–
Watchers 2 S	100	20	4
Veg.	25	0	0
Pretzels	110	0	1
Miracle Whip Free 2T	40	0	0
Milk	80	5	0
Supper			
Hamburger - lean	220	100	10
Bun	140	0	2
Veg. 2	50	0	0
Fries - lite	100	0	3
Soda	<u>150</u>	<u>0</u>	<u>0</u>
TOTALS	1660	130	23

Percent calories from fat--9 X 23 = 207 calories from fat divided by 1660 total calories = 12 percent calories from fat.
Exercise: type _____ time _____
Glasses of water: (8) _____

DAILY LOG   DATE ____/____/____   DAY 4
ALLOWED--Calories   1500   Fat (g) 33   20 percent
Cholesterol 150   Fat (g) 50   30 percent

Breakfast	Calories	CHOL.	Fat (g)
Coffee & sugar	15	0	0
Orange Juice 1/2 C	50	0	0
Shredded Wheat	110	0	0
Milk (nonfat) 1C	80	5	0
Any Fruit	40	0	0
Bread 1 S	70	0	1
Jelly 2t	35	0	0
Lunch			
Salad	100	0	0
S & W Free Dress. 3T	48	0	0
Almonds 1 oz. (10)	167	0	15
Ice tea + sugar	15	0	0
Any Fruit	40	0	0
Saltines 4	50	0	1
Cheese - Free	---	---	---
Philadelphia	50	10	0
Supper			
Spaghetti 1 C	155	0	1
Sauce - no meat	50	0	0
Mushrooms	25	0	0
Zucchini	25	0	0
Soda	150	0	0
Roll	100	0	1
Margarine 1 T	100	0	11
TOTALS	1475	15	30

Percent calories from fat--9 X 30 = 270 calories from fat divided by 1475 total calories = 18 percent calories from fat.
Exercise: type _____ time _____
Glasses of water: (8) _____

DAILY LOG　　　DATE _____/_____/_____　　DAY 5
ALLOWED--Calories　__1500__　　Fat (g) __33__　20 percent
Cholesterol __150__　　　　　　Fat (g) __50__　30 percent

Breakfast	Calories	CHOL.	Fat (g)
Coffee & sugar 15		0	0
Orange Juice 1/2 C.......................50		0	0
Quaker 100 % Natural....................110		0	2
Milk (nonfat) 1C...........................80		5	0
Any Fruit 40		0	0
Lunch			
McDonald's.................................-----		---	---
McLean Deluxe........................302		60	10
Fries - small..........................220		0	12
Soda 150		0	0
Supper			
Haddock 3.5 oz. 112		74	1
2 Veg...50		0	0
Milk..80		5	0
Roll..100		0	1
Ginger Snaps 3 90		0	2
Ice Cream - lite 1 C......................__90__		__5__	__3__
TOTALS................................. 1489		149	31

Percent calories from fat--9 X 31 = 279 calories from fat
divided by 1489 total calories = 18 percent calories from fat.
Exercise: type _____ time _____
Glasses of water: (8) _____

DAILY LOG   DATE _____/_____/_____   DAY 6
ALLOWED--Calories   1500   Fat (g) 33   20 percent
Cholesterol 150   Fat (g) 50   30 percent

Breakfast	Calories	CHOL.	Fat (g)
Coffee & sugar 15		0	0
Orange Juice 1/2 C.........................50		0	0
Pancakes ** 210		0	0
Strawberries or			
Blueberries 1C...........................100		0	0
Lunch			
Fruit Salad..................................120		0	0
Cheese 1 oz...............................110		28	9
Saltine 4 50		0	1
Soda 150		0	0
Tapioca **...................................85		2	0
Supper			
Ham Steak 3 oz. 122		45	4
Potato - large...............................100		0	0
Sour Cream -................................----		---	--
Fat Free - 2T..............................18		0	0
3 Veg...75		0	0
Roll...100		0	1
Margarine 1 T............................100		0	11
Ice Cream 1 C.............................90		5	3
TOTALS 1495		80	29

Percent calories from fat--9 X 29 = 261 calories from fat
divided by 1495 total calories = 17 percent calories from fat.
Exercise: type _____ time _____
Glasses of water: (8) _____
** See meal lists Chapter 29

DAILY LOG   DATE _____/_____/_____   DAY 7
ALLOWED--Calories   1500   Fat (g) 33   20 percent
Cholesterol 150   Fat (g) 50   30 percent

Breakfast	Calories	CHOL.	Fat (g)
Coffee & sugar 15		0	0
Orange Juice 1/2 C.......................50		0	0
French Toast 2 S........................140		0	2
Egg Beaters 1/2 C 50		0	0
Syrup - lite 3T *..........................240		0	0
Lunch			
Soup - many kinds 200		10	6
are below this.			
Bagel..150		0	1
Fruit - 2.......................................80		0	0
Cracker Jack...............................120		0	3
Supper			
Pork Chop...................................245		80	14
Corn on Cob..................................70		0	0
Baked Potato - small.......................70		0	0
Sour Cream -.............................. ---		---	---
Fat Free 2 T..................................18		0	0
Roll...100		0	1
Margarine 1 T............................100		0	11
TOTALS.................................. 1648		90	38

Percent calories from fat--9 X 38 = 342 calories from fat
divided by 1648 total calories = 21 percent calories from fat.
Exercise: type _____ time _____
Glasses of water: (8) _____
* Can use fresh fruit and save calories.

YOU CAN'T

GET MUCH DONE

BY STARTING

TOMORROW

CHAPTER 30

What About Cancer?

In 1989 the Surgeon General of The United States, C. Everett Koop, M.D., wrote the first Surgeon General's Report on Nutrition and Health.

The focus of his report was primarily on the relationship of diet to the occurrence of chronic diseases: coronary heart disease, high blood pressure, stroke, diabetes, obesity, and some types of cancer. I will concentrate here on what was in the report in regards to cancer.

The report stated that while many food factors are involved, chief among them is the over consumption of foods high in fat.

The report went on to say, it is now clear that diet contributes in substantial ways to the development of some cancers and that modification of diet can contribute to their prevention.

Some studies have found an association between overweight and increased risk for several cancers, especially cancer of the uterus and breast. There is also evidence that dietary fat increases the risk for cancer of the breast, colon, rectum, endometrium, and prostate.

Studies have also shown consistently that overall risk for death is increased with excess weight, with risk increasing as severity of obesity increases.

What can you do to reduce cancer risk factors? First, reduce fat consumption. I have discussed fat consumption throughout this book. You should know the percent of calories that come from fat in everything you eat. Use the appendices and the "Percent of Calories From Fat Chart." As you decrease fat, increase fiber in your diet.

Here are some ways to increase fiber.
1. Stuff a baked potato with broccoli for a fiber-rich dish that doesn't taste anything like bran. Both of those vegetable favorites rate high in fiber.
2. Snack on fiber-rich treats. Corn-bran cereal (Crunchy Bran) makes a perfect snack; it's quick, ready to eat, and can be kept in a jar at work. Other cereals like Wheat Chex and Bran Chex can be easily made into tasty snack mixes. Try mixing them with unsalted popcorn and chopped dried fruit to add more flavor and fiber.
3. Make your sweet tooth happy with fiber-rich fruits: apples, blackberries, raspberries, figs, prunes, and dates are all leaders on this count.
4. Substitute whole wheat flour for some of the white flour in recipes. Start by replacing about 1/3 of the white flour with whole wheat; increase to half whole wheat next time if the texture meets your approval. When baking, try whole wheat pastry flour.
5. Add beans to soups and salads—they have so much fiber that even small amounts can count. For those who won't touch beans, use peas—also a good source.
6. Crush whole-grain cereals, like shredded wheat or whole wheat flakes, with a rolling pin. Substitute for up to 1/3 of the flour in your favorite baked-goods recipe.
7. Use spoon-size shredded wheat, Wheat Chex, or Bran Chex cereals instead of croutons with soups and salads.
8. Discover the versatility of oats. Breakfast cereal and cookies are just the beginning. Oats also make a great extender for meats—for instance to replace bread crumbs in a meatloaf recipe. Quick oats also

make a great piecrust; use them instead of cracker crumbs.

9. Like oats, oat bran also has many uses. In addition to enjoying it as a hot cereal, you can sprinkle it on hot and cold foods or use it to replace some of the flour in baking. As you've been hearing, oat bran is rich in the type of fiber (water soluble) that helps to lower cholesterol.

10. Use All-Bran or 100% Bran Cereal to top cottage cheese, yogurt, and frozen desserts. Many people prefer the texture of these cereals to that of unprocessed bran.

11. Select coarse-grain foods like unprocessed bran and course textured crackers for the most laxative effect. These fiber sources don't have the cholesterol-lowering effect of foods like beans and oats, but appear to be the best choice for digestive health.

The Below Foods Are A Rich Sources of Fiber
4 grams or more

Cereals	serving 1 ounce	Legumes (cooked)	
All-Bran*,		Kidney, lima,	1/2 cup
Bran Buds*,		navy, pinto,	
100% Bran*,		white beans	
Bran Chex,			
Corn Bran,		**Fruits**	
Cracklin' Bran,		Blackberries	1/2 cup
40% Bran Flakes,		Dried prunes	3
raisin bran,			
Bran,	1/4 cup		
unprocessed*			
Wheat germ,	1 ounce		
toasted, plain			

Foods marked with an * have 6 grams or more of fiber per serving.

The Below Foods Are A Moderate Sources of Fiber
1 - 3 grams per serving

<u>Breads and Cereals</u>   Serving

Bran muffins   1 medium
Popcorn (air-popped)   1 cup
Whole wheat bread   1 slice
Whole wheat spaghetti   1 cup
Grape-Nuts, Most, shredded wheat, Total, Wheat Chex, Wheaties, granola- type and Cheerio-type cereals
Oatmeal, cooked   3/4 cup

<u>Legumes (cooked) and Nuts</u>

Chickpeas and lentils   1/2 cup
Almonds, peanuts   10 nuts

<u>Vegetables</u>

Artichoke   1 small
Asparagus, Green Beans,   1/2 cup
Brussels Sprouts, Cabbage,1/2 cup
Carrots, Cauliflower, Corn,
Peas, Kale, Parsnip,
Spinach (cooked or raw),
Squash, Turnip, Bean
Sprouts, Celery
Potato   1 medium
Sweet Potato   1/2 medium
Tomato   1 medium

<u>Fruits</u>

Apple   1 medium
Apricot, fresh   3 medium
Apricot, dried   5 halves
Banana   1 medium
Blueberries   1/2 cup
Cantaloupe   1/4 melon
Cherries   10
Dates, dried   3
Figs, dried   1 medium
Grapefruit   1/2
Orange   1 medium
Peach   1 medium
Pear   1 medium
Pineapple   1/2 cup
Raisins   1/4 cup
Strawberries   1 cup

What About Cancer?

The conclusion of Dr. Koop's Report is simple: increase fiber, decrease fat. Thirty-five percent of all cancer deaths may be related to what we eat. For more information on diet and cancer call the National Cancer Institute:
1-800-4-CANCER.

The "Percent of Calories From Fat Chart" contained in this book can help you lower your fat consumption.
Order one today for your refrigerator. See the coupon at the end of the book.

OBSTACLES

ARE THINGS YOU SEE

WHEN YOU TAKE

YOUR EYES

OFF THE

GOAL

CHAPTER 31

How Did You Get Here?

How does someone get overweight? A typical example is Jane. At 21 she felt great and was at her ideal weight. Five years later and not as active as when she was a teenager, her clothes feel tight and the scale has crept up five pounds. At 30 she has moved up one size in clothes and has added ten pounds. At 35 it's another size and another five pounds. The weight just sneaked up on her, 20 pounds in 14 years; that's less than one and a half pounds a year. Jane became overweight by not being as active as when she was a teenager but eating the same. I might add, this is what happened to me only I didn't gain weight. I weighed 175 pounds when I was eighteen and I weighed the same when I was forty but my waist was two inches bigger. You should know by now what happened. Slow inattention adds up to problems with weight. I lost some of my lean mass and replaced it with fat; and, fat takes up more space than lean mass. You can reverse this and weigh the same but fit into smaller clothes or lose weight if that's your goal.

Another case is Bob, who has always been heavy. In third grade he was 30 percent over his ideal weight; instead of weighing 50 pounds he weighed 65 pounds. At age 45 he is still 30 percent over his ideal weight, but now, instead of weighing 160 pounds he weighs 208 pounds. Unfortunately,

Bob has his parents to blame. His parents bought the groceries and made the meals during Bob's early years: plenty of meat, gravy, donuts, cookies, chips, and other items high in fat. Bob was sure to be getting over 40 percent of his calories from fat. In defense of his parents, they didn't know any better. But early family patterns act like an old map that hasn't been updated and needs to be for safe travel and sure direction. Bob's habits and tastes are firmly established but not unchangeable. Sometimes knowing how or why you got where you are helps you make changes.

Parents need to supervise what their children eat. Children can't be held responsible for knowing about nutrition. My kids would have a soda every night if I let them. In fact, they have a party almost every Friday night. They pick the supper: pizza, hot dogs, hamburgers, whatever. I know many Fridays they are getting over 30 percent of their calories from fat, but that's not the case the rest of the week.

Besides the weight accumulated through years or family patterns, certain preferences can control all the rest you do or eat.

Do you have a one item problem? A relative of mine does. She has five to eight servings of margarine a day. That's 500 to 800 calories and it is all 100 percent fat. She is an older woman and I would estimate her total calories should be around 1,200. She is getting a third or more of her calories from margarine. The rest of the things she eats are alright and if she reduced the margarine to one or two servings she would easily lose her excess 20 pounds. This adjustment is one of the easier ones to make, too.

One more example is Susan who had a baby. Five years later she is still blaming that baby for those 15 extra pounds. In fact, now it's 20. I would not tell anyone how much weight to gain while they are pregnant, that's for her doctor to do. But after the baby, if you follow this book, it will certainly help you lose weight.

Normally, you don't gain a lot of weight in a short time. Even in the last example, Susan ended up 20 pounds overweight after nine months. That's an average weight gain of about two pounds a month.

Perhaps one of these illustrations fits you? I know there are more examples but these are probably the most common. It doesn't matter how you ended up overweight. The solution is the same. Sneak up on your ideal weight through knowledge about foods you eat and make small habit changes. Lower your fat intake to less than 30 percent of your calories. The surefire, safe way to keep the weight off is to sneak it off one pound a week.

I am convinced that the overweight people and people with high cholesterol are getting over 30 percent of their calories from fat; the people with ideal weight and cholesterol are getting less than 30 percent of their calories from fat.

There is no easy way to lose weight, but it is easy to lose weight. There is no pill or magic potion that makes it easy to lose weight, but with the correct know-how it is easy to lose weight.

Your goal is to know the percent of fat, in terms of calories, in everything you eat; then make wise choices based on this knowledge.

Remember, a quick fix approach is a no-fix remedy. But, a slow fix plan is a sure success which can help produce a long healthy life.

THE PAST

CANNOT BE CHANGED;

THE FUTURE

IS STILL IN

YOUR POWER

CHAPTER 32

Last Words: Key Reminders

- One or two food items may be all that is keeping you from lower weight and cholesterol.

Cholesterol

- Almost no one with a cholesterol level below 160 develops heart disease. Lowering cholesterol may reverse the buildup in the arteries. Cholesterol levels over 200 are a health risk.
- Having your blood cholesterol level checked may uncover a problem long before it becomes serious, and if treated early, it may never become serious.
- Maintaining your ideal weight, and lowering your fat intake and cholesterol consumption will help lower your blood cholesterol level.

Exercise

- Increase the amount of physical activity in your daily routine. Use the stairs not the elevator.
- The best exercise is the one you enjoy.
- The exercise you choose should promote cardiovascular fitness. This allows the heart, lungs, and muscles the ability to process oxygen as efficiently as possible. As you become more fit and these components more efficient, your heart rate will drop. Your heart will accomplish the same thing at 55 beats per minute that it used to do at 72 beats.

- Walking is the most popular form of exercise.
- Stretches, warmup, and cool down are equally important in an exercise program if you want to avoid injury.
- Exercise will help you retain muscle and lose fat.

Don't Diet! Manage Your Food

- Permanent weight control is achieved by a well-balanced, lifetime eating plan based on a variety of foods that have maximum nutritional value. Small changes in lifestyle and eating habits can save you money and be healthier for you in the long run.
- If you eat the correct amount of carbohydrates, you will meet your body's glucose requirements. If you eat the correct amount of protein, you will meet your body's protein requirements. If you reduce your fat intake, your body will go after stored fat for muscle energy and leave the lean tissue alone.
- Carbohydrates, protein, and fat supply calories.
- Carbohydrates are absorbed into the bloodstream and stop hunger pangs faster than protein or fat.
- Carbohydrates supply glucose, a vital energy supply for your brain and nervous system.
- Carbohydrates and protein supply only 112 calories per ounce while fat supplies 252 calories per ounce.
- Food protein's first role is to replenish body protein. Too much protein can be dangerous.
- Various diets or eating programs can cause you to lose water, muscle, or fat.
- A diet that causes you to lose muscle (lean tissue) can result in a lot of weight loss, but it will be detrimental to your health.

Calories

- Remember, calories are used in three ways: ·
    1. digesting food
    2. physical activity
    3. basal metabolic rate (BMR).

Approximately 65 percent of the calories consumed in a day are used to supply the energy for the basic work of the body's cells to maintain life (basal metabolic rate). Lean tissue requires more calories for your BMR 24 hours a day. It's the calorie demand of your BMR that keeps the fat people fat and the thin people thin.

172

- If you consume more calories than you burn, the extra calories are stored as fat. This storage is unlimited.

Fat

- Saturated fat raises cholesterol levels more than anything else you eat.
- According to the U.S. Government:
    1. About one-third of all cancer deaths may be related to what we eat.
    2. A diet low in total fat may reduce the risk for cancers of the breast, prostate, colon, and rectum.
- Americans average 42 percent of their calories from fat. It's no wonder as a nation we are overweight. Fat is less filling than carbohydrates, provides energy slower, and has many more calories. Fat consumption should be less than 30 percent of energy intake if you want to control weight and cholesterol.
- You can not obtain 40 percent or more of your calories from fat and expect to lose weight or lower cholesterol. You need to know the percent of calories that are derived from fat in everything you eat.
- Like tobacco and alcohol addiction, some people are addicted to fat and don't know it. But fat addiction is the easiest of the three to beat. Most people think a candy bar is all sugar. Think again—most are 40 to 60 percent fat! Your taste buds can change but the key is to know the percent of fat in everything you eat.
- Using the "PERCENT OF CALORIES FROM FAT CHART" in this book can help you to consume less fat.
- The "PERCENT OF CALORIES FROM FAT CHART" is the cornerstone to good eating habits and weight control. This information is vital to good health. Use the chart often. With this knowledge you will succeed. Good luck on your new venture to lead a healthier, happier, longer life.

FOOD SUPPLY - ENERGY SOURCE - This flow chart shows what happens to each energy source as it enters your body.

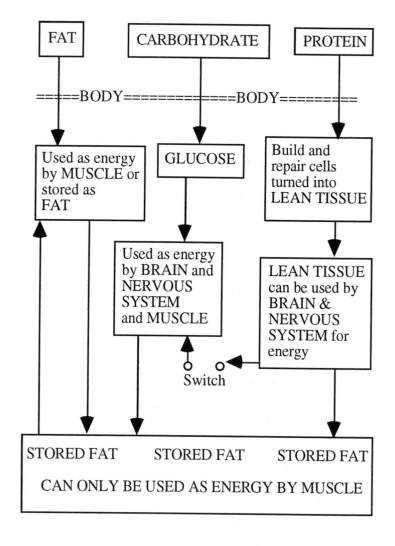

_ Your internal switch will use LEAN TISSUE to supply energy for your BRAIN and NERVOUS SYSTEM, if you are on a low calorie diet. You want to avoid this lean tissue loss. You avoid this lean tissue loss by limiting fat to less than 30 percent of total calories. Twenty percent would be just fine. Increase carbohydrates especially complex carbohydrates. Lose weight gradually; one pound a week. Your brain and nervous system consume more energy in a day than your muscles.

ACT

AS IF

IT WERE

IMPOSSIBLE

TO FAIL

CHAPTER 33

Motivation? - Go Have A Heart Attack

It's true. If you want to be motivated to lose weight and lower cholesterol, have a heart attack. The only problem with this drastic motivational technique is: only 25 percent survive heart attacks. These are not the kind of odds I would want if I had my choice. If you have survived a heart attack it is a blessing and it is not in disguise. A friend of my mother's had a heart attack and triple bypass surgery some time ago. Now in his 80's, he walks and rides an exercise bike and watches what he eats. He could pass for a man in his 60's.

A co-worker of mine, in his early 40's and at least 70 pounds overweight, needed to have angioplasty. He never had a heart attack or even chest pains, but during a routine EKG an irregular tracing led to the balloon procedure that opens arteries. After the procedure he never lost any of the weight even though he had heart disease and high blood pressure. When I was going through my recovery and losing weight, along with lowering my cholesterol, he said, "You know, I never had a heart attack, and that's why I'm not motivated like you." Maybe that was true for him. Possibly the doctors didn't stress the urgency for him to make some changes. Whatever the reason, he was not motivated.

I know firsthand why I was motivated. I still remember being curled up like a ball on the floor of the emergency room and feeling like an elephant was standing on my chest. Not something I'd care to go through again, and I surely wouldn't recommend it as a way to get motivated. This experience encouraged me to find out all I could about heart disease and what I could do, so it wouldn't happen again.

Motivation comes in two types: positive and negative. I have taught at the college and professional level, and I have been a flight instructor for over 20 years. Both positive and negative motivation are used in education and business, but both may not work for you. Once again, the key is: we are individuals. What motivates one person may not motivate another. The examples that follow won't motivate everyone. After all, scores of books have been written dealing with motivation. Hopefully, you will find one thing you can hang your hat on. The least you should get from this chapter is— whether you want to lose weight or lower cholesterol, you need to be motivated.

If you have high cholesterol, high blood pressure, a weight problem, or heart disease, you may be motivated into action. I know one person whose father and brother had heart attacks at an early age. It was after his brother's heart attack that he started to take his health seriously. This is a prime example of negative motivation: taking action because you're afraid something bad might happen to you.

I know one lady who thought she would feel better if she lost some weight and started to exercise. She started her program just being motivated by the idea she wanted to have more pep and energy. Her program got a real boost (positive) one day when she fit into a pair of slacks she hadn't been able to wear in two years. Numerous people said she looked great. Don't you think that gave her a lift! And she found she did have more pep and energy. All were forms of positive motivation.

You should think of some things to motivate you. I thought, "I'm too smart to die of a heart attack at 41 just because I don't know enough to take care of my health."

A good idea is to write down some goals. Tell yourself you can do it and have a positive attitude. Whether you want to lose weight or lower cholesterol write down what you want to do to achieve success. It's been proven over and over that people who write down specific steps have a far better chance to succeed than those who don't. Write your goals in the present tense as though they already exist. Read or write them every day. Post them on the bathroom mirror or anywhere else that will help you stay on track.

These goals will help you lose weight safely and easily.

STEPS:

1. I will increase my knowledge about nutrition.
2. I will keep a list of things I eat.
3. I will watch for foods high in fat.
4. I will substitute foods low in fat.
5. I will then get to eat more.

Know what your goals are and map out a plan of action that will lead you to that end.

EXAMPLES OF GOALS WRITTEN IN PRESENT TENSE:

1. I have lost 20 pounds in 25 weeks.
2. I fit into a size _____.
3. My cholesterol has gone down to _____.

Don't give up if you slip. Successful people make mistakes but they don't give up. They deal with the mistakes to correct them rather than pretend they didn't happen. So admit you slipped, then get on with how you can correct the problem. Above all, don't dwell on the mistake or feel guilty. I'll tell you right now, you are going to eat some things you will later feel you shouldn't have eaten. Think about what you might eat next time in place of that item, then move forward and don't look back.

If you come across a saying that sticks in your mind and motivates you, paste it on your bathroom mirror and read it everyday. "Nothing tastes as good as being fit feels." "I've been heavy and I've been light; believe me light is better."

The word lifestyle has been used a number of times in this book. What does it mean? It means what you do; it's unique to you, the individual. It's all your habits put together, and habits are just learned behaviors. Habits can be unlearned or changed. In regards to eating, a habit could be putting salt on your food before you ever taste it. Once you are aware of what you are eating, it may take a little conscious effort to change a habit that is unhealthy. Most habits can be changed in one week. Try it. See if I'm not right. Pick an eating habit you want to change, and work at it for one week. After that week it should be automatic. This may seem unimportant, but it's these very eating habits and motivation that are the cornerstones of your success.

Here's a good habit. Drink a glass of water before every meal. Everyone should have eight glasses of water a day. This includes the water in soda and juice drinks. I recommend you have at least four glasses of plain water every day. You could start a habit of one glass with each meal and one each time you brush your teeth. Water is critical to good health. Remember it's one of the six essential nutrients. In fact, it is the most important one.

Water has many functions:
1. Washes out toxic wastes
2. Regulates body temperature
3. Helps maintain the correct volume and pressure of your blood
4. Lubricates your joints and much more ...

Some people are going to say, "Wait a minute, I retain water so I have to cut back on how much I drink." They may even take a diuretic. Wrong! The best diuretic there is, is water. If you try to consume less water your body will try to conserve water. If your doctor has you on a diuretic, be honest with him and tell him how much water you drink in a day.

NOTE: Some conditions do require you to consume less water. Make sure you discuss this with your doctor and you understand what is right for you.

I may have initially started my program because of negative motivation (fear of having another heart attack) but positive motivation soon joined hands. The knowledge I gained seemed to inspire me to succeed. The loss of one pound a week, just as my dietitian predicted, gave me positive feedback to move forward. Watching my weight and cholesterol go down, eliminating back ache, sleeping better, having more energy, and feeling better all round are just a few of the positive reasons you will be successful with this plan.

I can virtually guarantee if you follow the guidelines in this book for 37 days, it will help you lose weight easily and safely. Many of you will no longer have high cholesterol or high blood pressure. The ease at which results are obtained will astound you.

Are you motivated to try this program for 37 days? Can you trade some unhealthy habits for healthy ones? I can't do it for you. I can provide the information. You may have to read the book as many times as it takes for that information to become applicable knowledge. That means you remember it or at least can find it quickly. Make it your hobby. I can think of no other hobby that will give you the rewards that good health will. You can do it. The key is having knowledge. I hope my heart attack will save YOUR life.

NOTHING

TASTES AS GOOD

AS BEING FIT

FEELS

CHAPTER 34

Eight Key Things To Remember

1. PLAN all MEALS. Don't just eat.
2. KNOW the PERCENT of CALORIES that come FROM FAT in everything you eat. Use the percent of fat chart.
3. DRINK 6 to 10 (8 ounce) glasses of WATER a day. One each time you brush your teeth and one before each meal. Water helps in metabolizing body fat.
4. Eat THREE OR MORE SERVINGS of FRUIT each day. This should be fresh fruit or dried fruit, not canned fruit because canned fruit has added sugar. One exception you may have is canned pineapple, which usually has no added sugar— read the label.
5. Eat THREE OR MORE SERVINGS of VEGETABLES; raw, steamed, or sauté—use any common seasoning (watch the salt). When you sauté use a non-stick pan and cooking spray. ** Do not use butter, oil, margarine, or any other fat or grease.
6. Eat SIX OR MORE SERVINGS of the BREAD, CEREAL, RICE, and PASTA GROUP. These

items should only have one or two grams of fat per serving. Give preference to whole grain products.

NOTE: Up to this point you will have consumed only between six and twelve grams of fat. From here on you have to watch the fat.

7. Eat TWO TO THREE SERVINGS of MILK, or MILK PRODUCTS. Choose LOW-FAT OR NO-FAT items. Watch the fat.

8. Eat a MAXIMUM of two to three servings of lean meat, poultry, eggs, or fish. About SIX OUNCES is the MAXIMUM TOTAL MEAT IN A DAY. Try to have one or two days a week where you eat none of these. Fish is a first choice and poultry second. You may have beans in place of meat but watch the added fat. You may have peanut butter in moderation: two tablespoons count as one ounce of lean meat.

You cannot be your ideal weight if 40 percent or more of your calories come from fat. You will not be overweight if twenty percent or less of your calories come from fat. It is just that simple. You should be somewhere between these figures: If 20 percent of your calories come from fat you will lose weight, if no more than 30 percent come from fat you will be able to maintain your weight. These rules will hold true for most people.

GOOD HEALTH
JUST DOESN'T TAKE
CARE OF ITSELF, AND
IT IS MOST OFTEN LOST
BY ASSUMING THAT IT WILL

CHAPTER 35

Hooray For Oprah Winfrey

She did it! You can too!

This book was in the final stages when Oprah Winfrey divulged how she lost all her weight after a thirteen year struggle. On her show in Nov. of 1993 she told all. I knew she had lost weight and I was in the process of editing the places in this book where I had mentioned her. I decided not to delete them even though they referred to her rapid weight loss in 1988 when she was unsuccessful. This time, however, it looks like she did it correctly.

On her Nov. 93 show, Oprah seemed so relaxed, uninhibited and at peace with herself. I was thoroughly impressed. She had kept a diary throughout her weight loss in 1988 up to this show. I wish everyone who is overweight could have seen this show; it was that good!

During this show she presented statistics from both of her weight loss programs. She not only kept track of her weight each week, but also she knew the percent of body fat, lean tissue lost, and fat lost. THESE FIGURES FURTHER SUBSTANTIATE SEVERAL THINGS THAT I'VE STATED IN THIS BOOK.

Let's take a look at the figures from each of the weight loss programs and compare the differences.

The two charts show the date, what she weighed, what her percent of body fat was, and goes on to show how much lean tissue was lost that month and how much fat was lost along with the total weight lost and what was the average weight lost per/week. I will explain the charts more as you read on.

In July of 1988 Oprah began a nationally known liquid diet under a doctor's supervision. She did not eat solid food for four months. Below are the results of that program.

FIRST PROGRAM - 1988

DATE	WEIGHT	PERCENT BODY FAT	LEAN TISSUE LOST	FAT LOST	POUNDS LOST	AVERAGE PER/WK.
July	212 lb.	38%	------- Start Program -------			
Aug.	192 lb.	35%	6 lb	14	20	5
Sept.	175 lb.	33%	8	9	17	4.2
Oct.	160 lb.	30%	5	10	15	3.7
Nov.	145 lb.	28%	7	7	14	3.7
TOTALS			26	40	66	4.1

RESULTS

Total weight lost - 66 pounds in four months.
Average 4.1 pounds per/week.
Total lean tissue lost - 26 pounds.
Total fat tissue lost - 40 pounds.

In March 1993 she started a new program. She took as much fat as possible out of her diet and she started to exercise. She ate regular food but less than 30 percent of her calories came from fat; she thinks about 20 percent came from fat. Below are the results of this program.

SECOND PROGRAM - 1993

DATE	WEIGHT	PERCENT BODY FAT	LEAN TISSUE LOST	FAT LOST	POUNDS LOST	AVERAGE PER/WK.
Mar.	222 lb.	41%	------- Start Program -------			
May	195 lb.	35%	4	23	27	3.3
July	177 lb.	30%	3	15	18	2.2
Sept.	161 lb.	25%	3	13	16	2.0
Nov.	150 lb.	20%	1	10	11	1.3
TOTALS			11	61	72	2.2

RESULTS
Total weight lost - 72 pounds in eight months.
Average 2.2 pounds per/week.
Total lean tissue lost - 11 pounds.
Total fat tissue lost - 61 pounds.

What do these figures reveal? What can they prove? In her 1988 program she lost over four pounds a week and got down to 145 pounds but her body fat was at 28 percent and she lost far too much lean tissue (26 pounds). If you lose lean tissue you will have to stay on a low calorie consumption diet to keep your weight down. Remember, your metabolic rate is directly affected by your ratio of body fat to lean tissue (Chap. 16).

The ideal percent of body fat for women is about 20 percent. Women with more than 30 percent body fat are considered obese (Chap.17). Oprah was at her ideal weight of 145 pounds; yet, with 28 percent body fat she was very close to being obese. If you had seen how thin she looked at the end of the first weight loss program in 1988 I doubt that you would have guessed she was close to being obese. I don't think she thought she was but, she did indeed have too much body fat. Remember, excess body fat has been linked to such health problems as coronary heart disease, high blood pressure, osteoporosis, diabetes, arthritis and certain forms of cancer (Chap. 17).

On her second program in 1993 she averaged only 2.2 pounds lost per/week over eight months. She lost more weight the second time (72 pounds) than the first time (66 pounds). More importantly, she lost less of the weight in lean tissue: only 11 pounds compared to 26 pounds. And, at the end of her second program she had attained 20 percent body fat. (Female athletes average 12 to 18 percent body fat. Chap. 17)

If you look at the last month of each program you will see something shocking. Notice the fat loss and lean tissue loss for Nov. 88. Seven pounds for each! That's one pound of lost lean tissue for one pound of lost fat! — or, a ratio of one to one! That's not just bad, it's dangerous. Please, for your own good health do not stay on any program that results in this kind of ratio.

Compare that to Nov. 1993: one pound of lean tissue to ten pounds of fat. This is great! It's a ratio of one to ten. Also, in her second program the lean tissue loss steadily decreased from four pounds to one pound. Remember, you do not want to lose lean tissue (Chaps. 16, 18). You want to keep lean tissue loss to a minimum.

Look at the second program (1993) under the column "Average Per/wk." This represents the pounds she lost per/week over the two month period. You'll notice that as her average got closer to one pound per/wk., her amount of fat loss to lean tissue got better.

What does it all mean? In a rapid weight loss program your body can not get glucose from stored fat (fat can not be turned into glucose) and your body will break down lean tissue for glucose (Chaps. 7, 32).

KNOW THIS
1. If you burn more calories than you consume you will lose weight. Everyone knows this.
2. How much weight you lose depends on two things:
   A. How many calories your body needs to supply.
   B. Whether these body calories come from stored fat or lean tissue.

3. One pound of stored fat can supply 3,500 calories.
4. One pound of lean tissue can supply only 480 calories.

WITH THESE FOUR FACTS HERE IS AN EXAMPLE

If over the course of one week you burned 7,000 more calories than you ate, your body would have to supply the 7,000 calories from either stored fat, lean tissue, or a combination of the two. If you had a switch on your body and you could direct all the 7,000 calories to be taken from stored fat, you would lose 2 pounds (7,000 divided by 3,500—fact 3 above). If you put the switch on lean tissue, you would lose 14.5 pounds (7,000 divide by 480—fact 4 above). We don't have a real switch, but as you look at Oprah's two programs you can certainly see she had a great affect on whether she lost lean tissue or fat tissue.

Although you can lose weight faster by losing lean tissue this will hurt you in the long run. You will end up like Oprah after her first program; you will lose a lot of weight but not fat and you will have to continue on a low calorie diet. Any extra calories will go right to fat because there will be less lean tissue to burn them up.

Lean tissue uses more calories than fat tissue because lean tissue is more active metabolically than fat tissue. We need to keep our lean tissue. (Chaps. 16, 25)

Take a look at the two programs again. Pay close attention to the total lean tissue lost and the total fat tissue lost. Remember lean tissue is muscle and the heart is a muscle. Keep lean tissue loss to a minimum.

You can find out your percent of body fat by calling hospitals in your area and asking if they do a "Body Composition Analysis." Tell them you are interested in your percent of body fat. The cost in my area is 15 to 20 dollars. The local university in some cases will also offer this to the general public. A university will usually have facilities to determine percent of body fat for its athletes.

There are three methods commonly used to determine the percent of body fat and there may be some variance with the results. The three methods are: hydrostatic (weighing in water), electronic, and skinfold measurements.

The ideal for men is 15 percent, with male athletes between six to 12 percent (Chap. 17). My percent of body fat is 10 percent. I am sure that if Oprah keeps on her exercise program, she will see her percent of body fat approach the female athlete range of 12 to 18 percent. As her percent of body fat goes down, she will find she has to eat more or she will lose even more weight.

Remember this, if two people weigh the same but one has 20 percent body fat and the other has 40 percent body fat, the one with the lower body fat will get to eat more. Why? Because lean tissue uses more calories than fat tissue even while you sleep.

I know Oprah is eating more after her second program than after her first, because there was an eight percent difference in her percent of body fat. The main reason for her success is the fact that she has decreased the amount of fat she eats, thereby reducing the percent of calories that come from fat. You too can reduce fat consumption by using the "Percent of Calories From Fat Chart." This is truly the safest and surest way to reduce and maintain your weight. Just ask Oprah!

Your internal switch uses LEAN TISSUE or FAT to supply calories when not enough calories are consumed through food sources. This is an energy deficit.
Create a small energy deficit—200 to 500 calories per/day by reducing fat intake and adding light to moderate exercise.

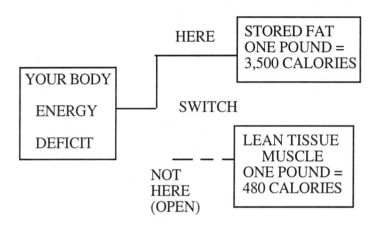

Keep your switch on STORED FAT by eating carbohydrates. If you cut back on carbohydrates your body switch will flip to lean tissue to get GLUCOSE because it can't get GLUCOSE from stored fat. This is just what happened to Oprah in her 1988 diet. Look at all the lean tissue she lost.

ONE

OF THE GREATEST

PLEASURES IN LIFE

IS DOING

WHAT PEOPLE SAY

YOU CANNOT DO

Appendix 1 Desirable Weights

(without shoes)   (without clothing)

Height	Weight		
MEN	Small	Medium	Large
5'1"	123-129	126-136	133-145
5'2"	125-131	128-138	135-148
5'3"	127-133	130-140	137-151
5'4"	129-135	132-143	139-155
5'5"	131-137	134-146	141-159
5'6"	133-140	137-149	144-163
5'7"	135-143	140-152	147-167
5'8"	137-146	143-155	150-171
5'9"	139-149	146-158	153-175
5'10"	141-152	149-161	156-179
5'11"	144-155	152-165	159-183
6'0"	147-159	155-169	163-187
6'1"	150-163	159-173	167-192
6'2"	153-167	162-177	171-197
6'3"	157-171	166-182	176-202

WOMEN	Small	Medium	Large
4'9"	99-108	106-118	115-128
4'10"	100-110	108-120	117-131
4'11"	101-112	110-123	119-134
5'0"	103-115	112-126	122-137
5'1"	105-118	115-129	125-140
5'2"	108-121	118-132	128-144
5'3"	111-124	121-135	131-148
5'4"	114-127	124-138	134-152
5'5"	117-130	127-141	137-156
5'6"	120-133	130-144	140-160
5'7"	123-136	133-147	143-164
5'8"	126-139	136-150	146-167
5'9"	129-142	139-153	149-170
5'10"	132-145	142-156	152-173
5'11"	135-148	145-159	155-176

SOURCE: Metropolitan Life Insurance Co.

Appendix 2: Meats

Fat and Cholesterol Comparison Chart
When following a cholesterol-lowering diet, select the meats that are lowest in saturated fat (i.e., saturated fatty acids) and cholesterol. The information on total fat, percent calories from fat, and calories should be helpful if you are trying to lose weight.

The following foods within each category (veal, lamb, beef, pork) are ranked from low to high saturated fat. To reduce the saturated fat in your diet, select the leaner cuts from the upper portion of each category. Trimming the visible fat will reduce the fat content even more. Since meats contribute a significant amount of saturated fat and cholesterol to your diet, you should eat smaller portions (no more than 6 ounces a day).

Product (3.5 Oz. Cooked)	Sat. Fat grams	Chol. mg.	Total Fat grams	Percent Calories From Fat	Total Calories
BEEF					
Kidneys, simmered	1.1	387	3.4	21	144
Liver, braised	1.9	389	4.9	27	161
Round, top round, lean only, broiled	2.2	84	6.2	29	191
Round, eye of round, lean only roasted	2.5	69	6.5	32	183
Round, tip round lean only, roasted	2.8	81	7.5	36	190
Round, full cut, lean only, choice, broiled	2.9	82	8.0	37	194
Round, bottom round, lean only, braised	3.4	96	9.7	39	222
Short loin, top loin, lean only, broiled	3.6	76	8.9	40	203
Wedge-bone sirloin, lean only, broiled	3.6	89	8.7	38	208

Appendix 2

Product (3.5 Oz. Cooked)	Sat. Fat grams	Chol. mg.	Total Fat grams	Percent Calories From Fat	Total Calories
Short loin, tender-loin lean only, broiled	3.6	84	9.3	41	204
Chuck, arm pot roast lean only, braised	3.8	101	10.0	39	231
Short loin, T-bone steak, lean only, choice, broiled	4.2	80	10.4	44	214
Short loin, porter-house steak, lean only, choice, broiled	4.3	80	10.8	45	218
Brisket, whole, lean only, braised	4.6	93	12.8	48	241
Rib eye, small end (ribs 10-12), lean only, choice, broiled	4.9	80	11.6	47	225
Rib, whole (ribs 6-12), lean only, roasted	5.8	81	13.8	52	240
Flank, lean only choice, braised	5.9	71	13.8	51	244
Rib, large end (ribs 6-9), lean only, broiled	6.1	82	14.2	55	233
Chuck, blade roast, lean only, braised	6.2	106	15.3	51	270
Corned beef, cured brisket, cooked	6.3	98	19.0	68	251
Flank, lean and fat, choice braised	6.6	72	15.5	54	257
Ground, lean, broiled medium	7.2	87	18.5	61	272
Round, full cut, lean and fat, choice, braised	7.3	84	18.2	60	274
Rib, short ribs, lean only, choice, braised	7.7	93	18.1	55	295

Appendix 2

Product (3.5 Oz. Cooked)	Sat. Fat grams	Chol. mg.	Total Fat grams	Percent Calories From Fat	Total Calories
Salami, cured, cooked, smoked, 3-4 slices	9.0	65	20.7	71	262
Short loin, T-bone steak, lean and fat, choice, broiled	10.2	84	24.6	68	324
Chuck, arm pot roast, lean and fat, braised	10.7	99	26.0	67	350
Sausage, cured, cooked, smoked, about 2	11.4	67	26.9	78	312
Bologna, cured, 3-4 slices	12.1	58	28.5	82	312
Frankfurter, cured, about 2	12.0	61	28.5	82	315
LAMB					
Leg, lean only, roasted	3.0	89	8.2	39	191
Loin chop, lean only, broiled	4.1	94	9.4	39	215
Rib, lean only, roasted	5.7	88	12.3	48	232
Arm chop, lean only, braised	6.0	122	14.6	47	279
Rib, lean and fat, roasted	14.2	90	30.6	75	368
PORK					
Cured, ham steak, boneless, extra lean, unheated	1.4	45	4.2	31	122
Liver, braised	1.4	355	4.4	24	165
Kidneys, braised	1.5	480	4.7	28	151
Fresh, loin, tenderloin, lean only, roasted	1.7	93	4.8	26	166
Cured, shoulder, arm picnic, lean only, roasted	2.4	48	7.0	37	170

Product (3.5 Oz. Cooked)	Sat. Fat grams	Chol. mg.	Total Fat grams	Percent Calories From Fat	Total Calories
Cured, ham, boneless, regular, roasted	3.1	59	9.0	46	178
Fresh, leg (ham), shank half, lean only, roasted	3.6	92	10.5	44	215
Fresh, leg (ham), rump half, lean only, roasted	3.7	96	10.7	43	221
Fresh, loin, center loin, sirloin, lean only, roasted	4.5	91	13.1	49	240
Fresh, loin, sirloin, lean only, roasted	4.5	90	13.2	50	236
Fresh, loin, center rib, lean only, roasted	4.8	79	13.8	51	245
Fresh, loin, top loin, lean only, roasted	4.8	79	13.8	51	245
Fresh, shoulder, blade, Boston, lean only, roasted	5.8	98	16.8	59	256
Fresh, loin, blade lean only, roasted	6.6	89	19.3	62	279
Fresh, loin, sirloin, lean and fat, roasted	7.4	91	20.4	63	291
Cured, shoulder, arm picnic, lean and fat, roasted	7.7	58	21.4	69	280
Fresh, loin, center loin, lean and fat, roasted	7.9	91	21.8	64	305
Cured, shoulder, blade roll, lean and fat, roasted	8.4	67	23.5	74	287
Fresh, Italian sausage-	9.0	78	25.7	72	323

Product (3.5 Oz. Cooked)	Sat. Fat grams	Chol. mg.	Total Fat grams	Percent Calories From Fat	Total Calories
Fresh, bratwurst, cooked	9.3	60	25.9	77	301
Fresh, chitterlings, cooked	10.1	143	28.8	86	303
Cured, liver sausage, liverwurst	10.6	158	28.5	79	326
Cured, smoked link sausage, grilled	11.3	68	31.8	74	389
Fresh, spareribs, lean and fat, braised	11.8	121	30.3	69	397
Cured, salami, dry or hard	11.9	- -	33.7	75	407
Bacon, fried	17.4	85	49.2	78	576
VEAL					
Rump, lean only, roasted	- -	128	2.2	13	156
Sirloin, lean only, roasted	- -	128	3.2	19	153
Arm steak, lean only, cooked	- -	90	5.3	24	200
Loin chop, lean only, cooked	- -	90	6.7	29	207
Blade, lean only, cooked	- -	90	7.8	33	211
Cutlet, medium fat, braised or broiled	4.8	128	11.0	37	271
Foreshank, medium fat, stewed	- -	90	10.4	43	216
Plate, medium fat, stewed	- -	90	21.2	63	303
Rib, medium fat, roasted	7.1	128	16.9	70	218
Flank, medium fat, stewed	- -	90	32.3	75	390

NOTES:

3.5 oz. = 100 grams (approximately)

Total Fat = Saturated fatty acids plus monounsaturated fatty acids plus polyunsaturated fatty acids.

Percent calories from fat = (total fat calories divided by total calories) multiplied by 100; total fat calories = total fat (grams) multiplied by 9.

Liver and most organ meats are low in fat, but high in cholesterol. If you are eating to lower your blood cholesterol, you should consider your total cholesterol intake before selecting an organ meat.

-- = information not available in the source used.

Appendix 3: Poultry

Fat and Cholesterol Comparison Chart
When following a cholesterol-lowering diet, select poultry low in saturated fat (i.e., saturated fatty acids) and cholesterol. Choosing poultry lower in total fat, calories, and percent calories from fat will also help you lose weight.

This table ranks poultry from low to high in saturated fat. Select the lower fat poultry from the upper portion of the table. In general, poultry, especially poultry with the skin removed, is lower in saturated fat than most cuts of meat. To reduce the saturated fat in your diet even more, eat smaller servings (no more than 6 ounces a day).

Product (3.5 Oz. Cooked)	Sat. Fat grams	Chol. mg.	Total Fat grams	Percent Calories From Fat	Total Calories
Turkey, fryer, roasters light meat without skin, roasted	0.4	86	1.9	8	140
Chicken, roasters, light meat without skin, roasted	1.1	75	4.1	24	153
Chicken, broilers or fryers, light meat without skin, roasted	1.3	85	4.5	24	173
Turkey, fryer- roasters, dark meat without skin, roasted	1.4	112	4.3	24	162
Chicken, stewing, light meat without skin, stewed	2.0	70	8.0	34	213
Turkey roll, light and dark	2.0	55	7.0	42	149
Turkey, fryer- roasters, dark meat with skin, roasted	2.1	117	7.1	35	182

Product (3.5 Oz. Cooked)	Sat. Fat grams	Chol. mg.	Total Fat grams	Percent Calories From Fat	Total Calories
Chicken, roasters, dark meat without, skin, roasted	2.4	75	8.8	44	178
Chicken, broilers or fryers, dark meat without skin, roasted	2.7	93	9.7	43	205
Chicken, broilers or fryers, light meat with skin, roasted	3.0	85	10.9	44	222
Chicken, stewing, dark meat without skin, stewed	4.1	95	15.3	53	258
Duck, domesticated, flesh only, roasted	4.2	89	11.2	50	201
Chicken, broilers or fryers, dark meat with skin, roasted	4.4	91	15.8	56	253
Goose, domesticated, flesh only, roasted	4.6	96	12.7	48	238
Turkey bologna, about 3 & 1/2 slices	5.1	99	15.2	69	199
Chicken frankfurter, about 2	5.5	101	19.5	68	257
Turkey frankfurter, about 2	5.9	107	17.7	70	226

NOTES:

3.5 oz. = 100 grams (approximately)

Total Fat = Saturated fatty acids, plus monounsaturated fatty acids, plus polyunsaturated fatty acids.

Percent calories from fat = (total fat calories divided by total calories) multiplied by 100; total fat calories = total fat (grams) multiplied by 9.

Appendix 4: Fish and Shellfish

Fat and Cholesterol Comparison Chart
When following a cholesterol-lowering diet, you may want to eat more fish and shellfish, which in general have a lot less saturated fat (i.e., saturated fatty acids) and cholesterol than meat and poultry. However, some shellfish is relatively high in cholesterol and should be eaten less often. Fish and shellfish also contain less total fat and calories than meat and poultry. Use the information on total fat, percent calories from fat, and calories to help you lose weight.

This table ranks fish and shellfish within each category (finfish, crustaceans, mollusks) from low to high in saturated fat. You will want to select the lower fat and cholesterol fish and shellfish from the upper portion of the table. To reduce the amount of saturated fat in your diet even more, eat smaller portions (no more than 6 ounces a day).

Omega-3 fatty acid (fish oil) is a type of polyunsaturated fat found in the greatest amounts in fattier fish. Evidence is mounting that omega-3 fatty acids in the diet may help lower high blood cholesterol. Since their potential benefit is not fully understood, the use of fish oil supplements is not recommended. However, eating fish is beneficial because it not only contains omega-3 fatty acids but, more importantly, it is low in saturated fat.

Product (3.5 Oz. Cooked)	Sat. Fat grams	Chol. mg.	Total Fat grams	Percent Calories From Fat	Total Calories
FINFISH					
Haddock, dry heat	0.2	74	0.9	7	112
Cod, Atlantic, dry heat	0.2	55	0.9	7	105
Pollock, walleye, dry heat	0.2	96	1.1	9	113
Perch, mixed species, dry heat	0.2	42	1.2	9	117
Grouper, mixed species, dry heat	0.3	47	1.3	10	118
Whiting, mixed species, dry heat	0.3	84	1.7	13	115

Product (3.5 Oz. Cooked)	Sat. Fat grams	Chol. mg.	Total Fat grams	Percent Calories From Fat	Total Calories
Snapper, mixed species, dry heat	0.4	47	1.7	12	128
Halibut, Atlantic/ Pacific, dry heat	0.4	41	2.9	19	140
Rockfish, Pacific, dry heat	0.5	44	2.0	15	121
Sea bass, mixed species, dry heat	0.7	53	2.5	19	124
Trout, rainbow, dry heat	0.8	73	4.3	26	151
Swordfish, dry heat	1.4	50	5.1	30	155
Tuna, bluefin, dry heat	1.6	49	6.3	31	184
Salmon, sockeye, dry heat	1.9	87	11.0	46	216
Anchovy, European, canned	2.2	--	9.7	42	210
Herring, Atlantic, dry heat	2.6	77	11.5	51	203
Eel, dry heat	3.0	161	15.0	57	236
Mackerel, Atlantic, dry heat	4.2	75	17.8	61	262
Pompano, Florida, dry heat	4.5	64	12.1	52	211

CRUSTACEANS

Lobster, northern	0.1	72	0.6	6	98
Crab, blue, moist heat	0.2	100	1.8	16	102
Shrimp, mixed species, moist heat	0.3	195	1.1	10	99

MOLLUSKS

Whelk, moist heat	0.1	130	0.8	3	275
Clam, mixed species, moist heat	0.2	67	2.0	12	148
Mussel, blue, moist heat	0.9	56	4.5	23	172
Oyster, Eastern, moist heat	1.3	109	5.0	33	137

NOTES:

3.5 oz. = 100 grams (approximately)

Total Fat = Saturated fatty acids, plus monounsaturated fatty acids, plus polyunsaturated fatty acids.

Percent calories from fat = (total fat calories divided by total calories) multiplied by 100; total fat calories = total fat (grams) multiplied by 9.

-- = information not available in sources used.

Appendix 5: Dairy and Egg products

Fat and Cholesterol Comparison Chart
When following a cholesterol-lowering diet, select dairy products low in saturated fat (i.e., saturated fatty acids) and cholesterol. Whole milk dairy products are relatively high in both when compared ounce for ounce with meat, poultry, and seafood. If you are trying to lose weight on your cholesterol-lowering diet, choose dairy products low in total fat, calories, and percent calories from fat.

The following foods within each category (milk, yogurt, cheese) are ranked from low to high in saturated fat. In general, the hard cheeses are much higher in saturated fat and cholesterol than yogurt and most soft cheeses. You will want to select foods from the upper portion of each category.

Product	Sat. Fat grams	Chol. mg.	Total Fat grams	Percent Calories From Fat	Total Calories
MILK (8 ounces)					
Skim milk	0.3	4	0.4	5	85
Buttermilk	1.3	9	2.2	20	99
Low-fat milk, 1% fat	1.6	10	2.6	23	102
Low-fat milk, 2% fat	2.9	18	4.7	35	121
Whole milk, 3.3% fat	5.1	33	8.2	49	150
YOGURT (4 ounces)					
Plain yogurt, low fat	0.1	2	0.2	3	63
Plain yogurt	2.4	14	3.7	47	70
CHEESE					
Cottage cheese, low-fat, 1% fat, 4 oz.	0.7	5	1.2	13	82
Mozzarella, part-skim, 1 oz.	2.9	16	4.5	56	72
Cottage cheese, creamed, 4 oz.	3.2	17	5.1	39	117
Mozzarella, 1 oz.	3.7	22	6.1	69	80
Sour cream, 1 oz.	3.7	12	5.9	87	61
American processed cheese spread, pasteurized, 1 oz.	3.8	16	6.0	66	82
Feta, 1 oz.	4.2	25	6.0	72	75

Product	Sat. Fat grams	Chol. mg.	Total Fat grams	Percent Calories From Fat	Total Calories
Neufchatel, 1 oz.	4.2	22	6.6	81	74
Camembert, 1 oz.	4.3	20	6.9	73	85
American processed cheese food, pasteurized, 1 oz.	4.4	18	7.0	68	93
Provolone, 1 oz.	4.8	20	7.6	68	100
Limburger, 1 oz.	4.8	26	7.7	75	93
Brie, 1 oz.	4.9	28	7.9	74	95
Romano, 1 oz.	4.9	29	7.6	63	110
Gouda, 1 oz.	5.0	32	7.8	69	101
Swiss, 1 oz.	5.0	26	7.8	65	107
Edam, 1 oz.	5.0	25	7.9	70	101
Brick, 1 oz.	5.3	27	8.4	72	105
Blue, 1 oz.	5.3	21	8.2	73	100
Gruyere, 1 oz.	5.4	31	9.2	71	117
Muenster, 1 oz.	5.4	27	8.5	74	104
Parmesan, 1 oz.	5.4	22	8.5	59	129
Monterey Jack, 1 oz.	5.5	25	8.6	73	106
Roquefort, 1 oz.	5.5	26	8.7	75	105
Ricotta, part-skim, 4 oz.	5.6	25	9.0	52	156
American processed cheese, pasteurized, 1 oz.	5.6	27	8.9	75	106
Colby, 1 oz.	5.7	27	9.1	73	112
Cheddar, 1 oz.	6.0	30	9.4	74	114
Cream cheese, 1 oz.	6.2	31	9.9	90	99
Ricotta, whole milk 4 oz.	9.4	58	14.7	67	197
EGGS					
Egg, chicken, white	0	0	tr.	0	16
Egg, chicken, whole	1.7	274	5.6	64	79
Egg, chicken, yolk	1.7	272	5.6	80	63

NOTES:
Total Fat = Saturated fatty acids, plus monounsaturated fatty acids, plus polyunsaturated fatty acids.
Percent calories from fat = (total fat calories divided by total calories) multiplied by 100; total fat calories = total fat (grams) multiplied by 9.
oz. = ounce
tr. = trace

Appendix 6: Frozen Desserts

Fat and Cholesterol Comparison Chart
When following a cholesterol-lowering diet, select frozen desserts low in saturated fat (i.e., saturated fatty acids) and cholesterol. This table ranks frozen desserts from low to high in saturated fat. Select the lower fat desserts from the upper portion of the list. If you are also trying to lose weight on your cholesterol-lowering diet, the calories will be of special interest to you. Although some frozen desserts are lower in fat than others, they may be just as high in calories as the higher fat products because of their sugar content. You will want to select those desserts not only low in fat but also low in calories.

Product (1 Cup)	Sat. Fat grams	Chol. mg.	Total Fat grams	Percent Calories From Fat	Total Calories
Fruit popsicle, 1	- -	- -	0.0	0	65
Fruit ice	- -	- -	tr.	0	247
Fudgsicle	- -	- -	0.2	2	91
Frozen yogurt, fruit flavored	- -	- -	2.0	8	216
Sherbet, orange	2.4	14	3.8	13	270
Pudding pops, 1 pop	2.5	1	2.6	25	94
Ice milk, vanilla, soft serve	2.9	13	4.6	19	223
Ice milk, vanilla, hard	3.5	18	5.6	28	184
Ice cream, vanilla, regular	8.9	59	14.3	48	269
Ice cream, french vanilla, soft serve	13.5	153	22.5	54	377
Ice cream, vanilla, rich, 16% fat	14.7	88	23.7	61	349

Appendix 7: Fats and Oils

Comparison Chart
This table compares the fat content of selected fats and oils, going from those with a low saturated fat (i.e., saturated fatty acids) content to those with a high saturated fat content. When following a cholesterol lowering diet, you will limit the amount of fat and oil in your diet. When necessary, use those fats which are lower in saturated fat, located in the upper portion of the table. All fats and oils are high in calories, 115-120 calories per tablespoon.

Product 1 Tablespoon	Sat. Fat grams	Chol. mg.	Polyun- saturated Fat grams	Monoun- saturated Fat grams
Rapeseed oil (canola oil)	0.9	0	4.5	7.6
Safflower oil	1.2	0	10.1	1.6
Sunflower oil	1.4	0	5.5	6.2
Peanut butter, smooth	1.5	0	2.3	3.7
Corn oil	1.7	0	8.0	3.3
Olive oil	1.8	0	1.1	9.9
Hydrogenated sunflower oil	1.8	0	4.9	6.3
Margarine, liquid, bottled	1.8	0	5.1	3.9
Margarine, soft, tub	1.8	0	3.9	4.8
Sesame oil	1.9	0	5.7	5.4
Soybean oil	2.0	0	7.9	3.2
Margarine, stick	2.1	0	3.6	5.1
Peanut oil	2.3	0	4.3	6.2
Cottonseed oil	3.5	0	7.1	2.4
Lard	5.0	12	1.4	5.8
Beef tallow	6.4	14	0.5	5.3
Palm oil	6.7	0	1.3	5.0
Butter	7.1	31	0.4	3.3
Cocoa butter	8.1	0	0.4	4.5
Palm kernel oil	11.1	0	0.2	1.5
Coconut oil	11.8	0	0.2	0.8

Appendix 8: Nuts and Seeds

Fat Comparison Chart
When following a cholesterol-lowering diet, You will be selecting foods low in saturated fat (i.e., saturated fatty acids) and cholesterol. This table ranks nuts and seeds from low to high in saturated fat. Choose those from the upper portion of the list. Most nuts and seeds would appear to be appropriate foods to eat because they contain little saturated fat. However, except for chestnuts, they are all high in total fat and consequently high in calories. Thus, if you are also trying to lose weight, you should limit the use of nuts and seeds in your diet.

Product 1 ounce	Sat. Fat grams	Chol. mg.	Total Fat grams	Percent Calories From Fat	Total Calories
European chestnuts	0.2	0	1.1	9	105
Filberts or hazelnuts	1.3	0	17.8	89	179
Almonds	1.4	0	15.0	80	167
Pecans	1.5	0	18.4	89	187
Sunflower seed kernels, roasted	1.5	0	14.0	77	165
English walnuts	1.6	0	17.6	87	182
Pistachio nuts	1.7	0	13.7	75	164
Peanuts	1.9	0	14.0	76	164
Hickory nuts	2.0	0	18.3	88	187
Pine nuts, pignolia	2.2	0	14.4	89	146
Pumpkin and squash seed kernels	2.3	0	12.0	73	148
Cashew nuts	2.6	0	13.2	73	163
Macadamia nuts	3.1	0	20.9	95	199
Brazil nuts	4.6	0	18.8	91	186
Coconut meat, unsweetened	16.3	0	18.3	88	187

Appendix 9: Breads, Cereals, Pasta, Rice, and Dried Peas and Beans

Fat and Cholesterol Comparison Chart
When following a cholesterol-lowering diet, You will be selecting foods low in saturated fat (i.e., saturated fatty acids) and cholesterol. To lose weight on your cholesterol-lowering diet, choose foods that are lower in total fat, percent calories from fat, and calories.

Each of the following categories (breads, cereals, pasta, rice, and dried peas and beans) is ranked from low to high in saturated fat. To reduce the saturated fat in your diet, select the products from the upper portion of each category.

Product	Sat. Fat grams	Chol. mg.	Total Fat grams	Percent Calories From Fat	Total Calories
BREADS					
Melba toast, 1 plain	0.1	0	tr.	0	20
Pita, 1/2 large shell	0.1	0	1.0	5	165
Corn tortilla	0.1	0	1.0	14	65
Rye bread, 1 slice	0.2	0	1.0	14	65
English muffin	0.3	0	1.0	6	140
Bagel, 1	0.3	0	2.0	9	200
White bread, 1 slice	0.3	0	1.0	14	65
Rye krisp, 2 triple crackers	0.3	0	1.0	16	56
Whole wheat bread, 1 slice	0.4	0	1.0	13	70
Saltines, 4	0.5	4	1.0	18	50
Hamburger bun	0.5	tr.	2.0	16	115
Hot dog bun	0.5	tr.	2.0	16	115
Pancake, 1 4" diameter	0.5	16	2.0	30	60
Bran muffin, 1, 2 & 1/2" diameter	1.4	24	6.0	43	125
Corn muffin, 1, 2 & 1/2" diameter	1.5	23	5.0	31	145
Plain doughnut, 1 3 & 1/4" diameter	2.8	20	12.0	51	210
Croissant, 1, 4 & 1/2" by 4"	3.5	13	12.0	46	235
Waffle, 1, 7" diameter	4.0	102	13.0	48	245

Product	Sat. Fat grams	Chol. mg.	Total Fat grams	Percent Calories From Fat	Total Calories
CEREALS (1 Cup)					
Corn flakes	tr.	- -	0.1	0	98
Cream of wheat, cooked	tr.	- -	0.5	3	134
Corn grits, cooked	tr.	- -	0.5	3	146
Oatmeal, cooked	0.4	- -	2.4	15	145
Granola	5.8	- -	33.1	50	595
100 % Natural Cereal with raisins and dates	13.7	- -	20.3	37	496
PASTA (1 Cup)					
Spaghetti, cooked	0.1	0	1.0	6	155
Elbow macaroni, cooked	0.1	0	1.0	6	155
Egg noodles, cooked	0.5	50	2.0	11	160
Chow mein noodles, canned	2.1	5	11.0	45	220
RICE (1 Cup cooked)					
Rice, white	0.1	0	0.5	2	225
Rice, brown	0.3	0	1.0	4	230
DRIED PEAS AND BEANS (1 Cup cooked)					
Split peas	0.1	0	0.8	3	231
Kidney beans	0.1	0	1.0	4	225
Lima beans	0.2	0	0.7	3	217
Black eyed peas	0.3	0	1.2	5	200
Garbanzo beans	0.4	0	4.3	14	269

Appendix 10: Sweets and Snacks

Fat and Cholesterol Comparison Chart
When following a cholesterol-lowering diet, select foods low in saturated fat (i.e., saturated fatty acids) and cholesterol. To lose weight on your cholesterol-lowering diet, see the information on total fat, percent fat, and calories. Since the foods in this table may be sweet, even if they are low in fat, they could be high in calories. Fruits, vegetables, and breads provide tasty, low-fat, low-calorie, alternatives.

The following foods within each category (beverages, candy, cookies, cakes and pies, snacks, and pudding) are ranked from low to high in saturated fat. To reduce the saturated fat in your diet, select the products from the upper portion of each category.

Product	Sat. Fat grams	Chol. mg.	Total Fat grams	Percent Calories From Fat	Total Calories
BEVERAGES					
Ginger ale, 12 oz.	0.0	0	0.0	0	125
Cola, regular, 12 oz.	0.0	0	0.0	0	160
Chocolate shake, 10 oz.	6.5	37	10.5	26	360
CANDY (1 ounce)					
Hard candy	0	0	0	0	110
Gum drops	tr.	0	tr.	tr.	100
Fudge	2.1	1	3.0	24	115
Milk chocolate, plain	5.4	6	9.0	56	145
COOKIES					
Vanilla wafers, 5 cookies, 1 & 3/4" diameter	0.9	12	3.3	32	94
Fig Bars, 4 cookies	1.0	27	4.0	17	210
Chocolate brownie with icing, 1 & 1/2" by 1 & 3/4" by 7/8"	1.6	14	4.0	36	100
Oatmeal cookies, 4 cookies, 2 & 5/8" diameter	2.5	2	10.0	37	245
Chocolate chip cookies 4 cookies 2&1/4" diameter	3.9	18	11.0	54	185

Product	Sat. Fat grams	Chol. mg.	Total Fat grams	Percent Calories From Fat	Total Calories
CAKE and PIES					
Angel food cake, _____ 1/12 of 10" cake	tr.	0	tr.	tr.	125
Gingerbread _____ 1/9 of 8" cake	1.1	1	4.0	21	175
White layer cake _____ with white icing, 1/16 of 9" cake	2.1	3	9.0	32	260
Yellow layer cake with _____ chocolate icing, 1/16 of 9" cake	3.0	36	8.0	31	235
Pound cake, _____ 1/17 of loaf	3.0	64	5.0	41	110
Devils food cake with _____ chocolate icing, 1/16 of 9" cake	3.5	37	8.0	31	235
Lemon meringue pie, _____ 1/6 of 9" pie	4.3	143	14.0	36	355
Apple pie, 1/6 of _____ 9" pie	4.6	0	18.0	40	405
Cream pie, 1/6 of _____ 9" pie	15.0	8	23.0	46	455
SNACKS					
Popcorn, air-popped _____ 1 cup	tr.	0	tr.	tr.	30
Pretzels, stick, 2&1/4" _____ 10 pretzels	tr.	0	tr.	tr.	10
Popcorn with oil _____ and salted, 1 Cup	0.5	0	3.0	49	55
Corn chips, 1 oz. _____	1.4	25	9.0	52	155
Potato chips, 1 oz. _____	2.6	0	10.1	62	147
PUDDING					
Gelatin _____	0.0	0	0.0	0	70
Tapioca, 1/2 Cup _____	2.3	15	4.0	25	145
Chocolate pudding, _____ 1/2 Cup	2.4	15	4.0	24	150

Appendix 11: Miscellaneous

Fat and Cholesterol Comparison Chart

	Sat. Fat grams	Chol. mg.	Total Fat grams	Percent Calories From Fat	Total Calories
GRAVIES (1/2 Cup)					
Au jus, canned	0.1	1	0.3	3	80
Turkey, canned	0.7	3	2.5	37	61
Beef, canned	1.4	4	2.8	41	62
Chicken, canned	1.7	3	6.8	65	95
SAUCES (1/2 Cup)					
Sweet & sour	tr.	0	0.1	<1	147
Barbecue	0.3	0	2.3	22	94
White	3.2	17	6.7	50	121
Cheese	4.7	26	8.6	50	154
Sour cream	8.5	45	15.1	53	255
Hollandaise	20.9	94	34.1	87	353
Bearnaise	20.9	99	34.1	88	351
SALAD DRESSINGS (1 Tablespoon)					
Russian, low calorie	0.1	1	0.7	27	23
French, low calorie	0.1	1	0.9	37	22
Italian, low calorie	0.2	1	1.5	85	16
Thousand Island, low calorie	0.2	2	1.6	59	24
Imitation mayonnaise	0.5	4	2.9	75	35
Thousand Island, regular	0.9	- -	5.6	86	59
Italian, regular	1.0	- -	7.1	93	69
Russian, regular	1.1	- -	7.8	92	76
French, regular	1.5	- -	6.4	86	67
Blue cheese	1.5	- -	8.0	93	77
Mayonnaise	1.6	8	11.0	100	99
OTHER					
Olives, green 4 medium	0.2	0	1.5	90	15
Nondairy creamer, powdered, 1 teaspoon	0.7	0	1.0	90	10
Avocado, Florida	5.3	0	27.0	72	340
Pizza, cheese, 1/8 of 15" diameter	4.1	56	9.0	28	290

Appendix 12 - CALORIES

1 Gram of Fat	equals 9 calories
1 Ounce of Fat	equals 252 calories
1 Gram of Protein	equals 4 calories
1 Ounce of Protein	equals 112 calories
1 Gram of Carbohydrate	equals 4 calories
1 Ounce of Carbohydrate	equals 112 calories

Fat takes 6 to 8 hours to burn up (nuts, olives, butter, veg. oil)

Protein takes 3 to 4 hours (meat, milk, eggs)

Carbohydrate, complex (starch) - (corn, potato, grain, peas, rice) take 1 to 2 hours

Carbohydrate, simple (sugar) - (fruit) take 15 to 45 minutes or less

Appendix 13 - QUALITY PROTEIN

For Quality Protein * from vegetable sources, use any food from column 1 in combination with a food from column 2.

	Column1	**Column2**
LEGUMES	<u>BEANS</u>: Adsuki, Black, Cranberry, Fava, Kidney, Limas, Pinto, Marrow, Mung, Navy, Pea, Soy, (Tofu) (Sprouts)	Low-fat dairy products
	<u>PEAS</u>: Black-eyed, Chick Cow, Field, Split LENTILS	Grains Nuts & Seeds
GRAINS	<u>WHOLE GRAINS</u>: Barley; Corn (cornbread) (grits) Oats; Rice; Rye, Wheat (Bulgur, Wheat Germ) Sprouts	Low-fat dairy products Legumes
NUTS & SEEDS	<u>NUTS</u>; Almonds, Beechnuts, Brazil nuts, Cashews, Filberts, Pecans, Pine nuts (Pignolia), Walnuts <u>SEEDS</u>: Pumpkin, Sunflower	Low-fat dairy products Legumes

* Low-fat dairy products (milk, yogurt, cheese, eggs, cottage cheese), in addition to being used as a supplement to the above, may be used alone as "quality protein."

Appendix 14 - Exchange System

The exchange system divides foods into six groups based on calories, proportions of carbohydrate, fat, and protein, and portion size. The groups along with the basic number of exchanges per day are shown on the table below. See Chapter Twelve for more information. The intent of the exchange system is to eat a variety of foods, so you obtain all the essential nutrients and still maintain your ideal weight. I only included a few foods in each list to give you an idea how they are grouped. You can add your own foods to each list, and it is possible to break down your favorite recipe to see how many exchanges it uses. Stay within the guidelines at the start of each list.

The table below shows the number of exchanges for various calorie intakes. The number of calories in one exchange is in parenthesis.

CALORIES per/day

Exchanges	1,000	1,200	1,500	1,800	2,000
Bread (70)	4	5	8	10	10
Vegetable (25)	2	3	3	3	4
Fruit (40)	3	4	4	5	5
Milk (80)	2	2	2	2	3
Lean Meat (55)	4	5	5	6	7
Fat (45)	4	5	6	7	8

The above table will supply about 30 percent of your total calories from fat. The fat contained in lean meat was taken into account; any other meat will decrease your fat exchanges.

How do you use this chart? If you decide you should have 1,500 calories per/day find 1,500 on the chart and go straight down. The first number you run into is eight which is across from bread; you are allowed eight bread exchanges. The next number is three across from vegetables, four across from fruit, two milk, five meat, and six fat. This is a total of 28 exchanges to be used each day.

It is important that you not go over your fat exchanges, but you could go under. In fact, you could trade one fat exchange for one fruit or two fat for one bread, keep the calories about even. But, you can't trade for extra fat exchanges. You can survive very nicely if only ten percent of your calories come from fat, so don't be afraid to give up some of the fat exchanges.

BREAD and STARCHY VEGETABLE LIST

One exchange is about equal to: 15 grams carbohydrate, 2 grams protein, and 70 calories. Check the Label.

Amount   Food

Bread
1 slice	White, Whole Wheat, Rye, Pumpernickel
1	Frankfurter or hamburger bun
1 half	Small bagel
1 half	Small English Muffin
1	Plain roll
1 6"	Tortilla

Cereal
1/2 C	Bran flakes
3/4 C	Ready to eat cereal, unsweetened
1/2 C	Cereal, cooked
1/2 C	Grits, cooked
1/2 C	White rice, wild rice, or barley, cooked
1/3 C	Brown rice, cooked
3 C	Popcorn, no fat added
3 Tbsp	Wheat Germ

Crackers
2	Graham, 2 & 1/2" square
Pretzels	70 calories worth
6	Saltines

Dried beans, peas, and lentils
1/2 C	Beans, peas, lentils, dried and cooked
1/4 C	Baked beans, no pork, canned - check fat content ratio to calories

Starchy Vegetables
1/3 C	Corn	
1	Corn on cob	
1/2 C	Lima beans	
1/2 C	Peas	
1 small	Potato	1/2 C Yam, Sweet Potato
3/4 C	Squash (Acorn, Butternut)	

VEGETABLE LIST

One exchange is about equal to: 5 grams carbohydrate, 2 grams protein, and 25 calories.

Amount	Food
all	
1/2 C	Artichoke
	Asparagus
	Beans (Green, Wax)
	Beets
	Cabbage
	Carrots
	Cauliflower
	Celery
	Cucumbers

Dark Green Vegetables
1/2 C	Beet greens
	Broccoli
	Collard greens
	Kale
	Mustard greens
	Spinach
	Turnip greens
	Eggplant
	Green pepper
	Mushrooms
	Rhubarb
	Sauerkraut
	Tomatoes or Juice
	Vegetable juice cocktail
	Zucchini

FRUIT LIST

One exchange is about equal to: 10 grams carbohydrate, and 40 calories.

Amount	Food
1 small	Apple
1/3 C	Apple juice
1/2 C	Applesauce
3	Apricots
1/2 Small	Banana
1/2 C	Blackberries
1/2 C	Blueberries
1/4 Small	Cantaloupe
1/2 C	Carrot juice
10 Large	Cherries
2	Figs
1/2	Grapefruit
1/2 C	Grapefruit juice
12	Grapes
1/4 C	Grape juice
1/8	Honeydew melon
1 small	Nectarine
1 small	Orange
1/2 C	Orange juice
1 medium	Peach
1 small	Pear
1/2 C	Pineapple
1/3 C	Pineapple juice
2 medium	Prunes
1/4 C	Prune juice
2 tbsp	Raisins
1/2 C	Raspberries
3/4 C	Strawberries
1 medium	Tangerine
1 C	Watermelon

MILK LIST - count other exchanges noted

One exchange is about equal to: 12 gram carbohydrate, 8 gram protein, no fat, and 80 calories. (A milk exchange is a serving of food equivalent to 1 cup of skim milk in its energy nutrient content.)

Amount   Food

Nonfat fortified milk
1C	Skim or nonfat milk
1C	Yogurt made from skim milk (plain)

Low-fat fortified milk
1C	1% fat fortified milk (count as 1 milk and 1/2 fat exchange
1C	2% fat fortified milk (count as 1 milk and 1 fat exchange) (contains 5 grams of fat)
1C	Yogurt made from 2% fortified milk (plain, unflavored) count as 1 milk and 1 fat.

Whole milk (count as 1 milk and 2 fat exchanges)
1C	Whole milk
1C	Buttermilk made from whole milk

Any product made from whole milk with 10 grams fat.

MEAT and MEAT ALTERNATE LIST

One exchange is about equal to: 7 grams protein, 3 grams fat, and variable added fat, 55 calories and extra calories for added fat. (A meat exchange is a serving of protein-rich food that contains negligible carbohydrate but a significant amount of protein (7 gram) and fat (3 gram), roughly equivalent to the amounts in 1 ounce of LEAN meat; contains about 55 calories.)

Amount	Food
Lean Meat - also check appendix 2.	
1 ounce	Beef, Lamb, Pork, Veal
1 ounce	Poultry - without skin
1 ounce	Fish
1/4 C	Canned salmon, tuna, mackerel, crab
1 ounce	Clams, oysters, scallops, shrimp
1 ounce	Cheese, made from skim milk
1/2 C	Dried beans and peas, cooked (count as 1 lean meat and 1 bread exchange)

Medium Fat Meat (count as 1 lean meat and 1/2 fat exchange

1 ounce	Beef - ground (15% fat),
1/4 C	Cottage cheese, creamed
1 ounce	Cheese - mozzarella, ricotta, farmer's cheese, Neufchatel, also check appendix 5
3 tbsp	Parmesan cheese
1	Egg (high in cholesterol)

High Fat Meat (count as 1 lean meat and 1 fat exchange) also check appendix 2.

1 ounce	Beef - ground (more than 20% fat), hamburger, (commercial), chuck (ground commercial)
1 ounce	Cheese, cheddar, also check appendix 5.
1 slice	Cold cuts, read label (see the chapter on label reading)
1 small	Frankfurter

Meat Alternates

2 tbsp	Peanut butter (count as 1 lean meat and 2 & 1/2 fat exchanges
4 tbsp	Peanuts (count as 1 lean meat, 1/2 bread, and 2 fat exchanges)

FAT LIST

One exchange is about equal to: 5 grams fat, and 45 calories.
Polyunsaturated fat

Amount	Food
1 tsp	Margarine (soft, tub or stick) check label
1 tsp	Oil - corn, safflower, sunflower, soy
1 tsp	Oil, Olive*
1 tsp	Oil, Peanut*
5 small	Olives*
10	Almonds* (see appendix 8)
2	Pecans*
Saturated fat	
1 tsp	Margarine, regular stick
1 tsp	Butter
2 tbsp	Cream, sour
1 tbsp	Cream cheese
1 tbsp	French dressing**
1 tbsp	Italian dressing**
1 tsp	Mayonnaise**
2 tsp	Salad dressing, mayonnaise type**

NOTES: * = Fat content is primarily monounsaturated
    ** = May be Polyunsaturated, check label

Appendix - 15

Food Label Weights and Measures

Weight
1 ounce (oz.) = approximately 28 grams (g)
16 ounces = 1 pound (lb)
1 pound = 454 grams
1 kilogram (kg) = 1,000 grams or 2.2 pounds
1 gram = 1,000 milligrams (mg)
1 milligram = 1,000 micrograms

Volume
1 liter = 1.06 quarts
1 liter = 1,000 milliliters (mL)
1 milliliter = 0.03 fluid ounces
1 gallon = 3.79 liters
1 quart = 0.95 liter
1 cup = 8 fluid ounces
1 tablespoon = 15 milliliters
3 teaspoons = 1 tablespoon
16 tablespoons = 1 cup
4 cups = 1 quart

Appendix 16 - Target Heart Rate

To find your target heart rate, subtract your age from 220 and then calculate 60 to 80 percent of that figure. Target heart rates have been figured and listed in the table below.

	TARGET HEART RATE	
AGE	60 percent	80 percent
20	120	160
25	117	156
30	114	152
35	111	148
40	108	144
45	105	140
50	102	136
55	99	132
60	96	128
65	93	124

E-Z-2 READ™
PERCENT OF CALORIES FROM FAT CHART™

Find the calories and grams of FAT per serving. Where the values intersect is how much of the serving is FAT. For example: **110** calories and **5** grams of fat = **41 % FAT.**

FAT grams	1	2	3	4	5	6	7	8	9	10	11
CALORIES											
60	15	30	45	60	75	90	**	**	**	**	**
70	13	26	39	51	64	77	90	**	**	**	**
80	11	23	34	45	56	68	79	90	**	**	**
90	10	20	30	40	50	60	70	80	90	**	**
100	9	18	27	36	45	54	63	72	81	90	**
110	8	16	25	33	41	49	57	65	74	82	90
120	8	15	23	30	38	45	53	60	68	75	83
130	7	14	21	28	35	42	48	55	62	69	76
140	6	13	19	26	32	39	45	51	58	64	71
150	6	12	18	24	30	36	42	48	54	60	66
200	5	9	14	18	23	27	32	36	41	45	50
250	4	7	11	14	18	22	25	29	32	36	40
300	3	6	9	12	15	18	21	24	27	30	33
350	3	5	8	10	13	15	18	21	23	26	28
400	2	5	7	9	11	14	16	18	20	23	25

** = Over 90 percent fat.

It is recommended that no more than 30 percent of your total calories come from fat.

NOTE: If you had numbers not on the chart, such as 500 calories and 20 grams of fat, you could divide each number by the same number to get back on the chart.

ORDER FROM: READERS CHOICE, 2141 Shaw Ave., Suite 1212, Clovis, CA. 93611-8916

$1 for plastic wallet size — plus self-addressed stamped envelope please. Great for the grocery store.

$3 for a magnetic-back chart that mounts on refrigerator size (4" by 6") — plus self-addressed stamped (2 ounces postage) and #10 envelope please.

Appendix - 18

TWENTY AND THIRTY PERCENT FAT CHART

The table below shows the amount of fat that provides between 20 and 30 percent of calories for diets of several total daily calorie intakes. After you determine how many calories you should be eating in a day, it is easy to select the right amount of fat. Then instead of keeping track of calories, keep track of grams of fat. Try to consume between the 20 and 30 percent figure for grams of fat.

Calories per/day	Amount of fat that provides 30 % calories	Amount of fat that provides 20 % calories
1,000	33 grams	22 grams
1,500	50 grams	33 grams
2,000	67 grams	44 grams
2,500	83 grams	55 grams
3,000	100 grams	66 grams

Appendix - 19 STRETCHES

1. Make circles with the head, rotating to the right and then to
   the left.

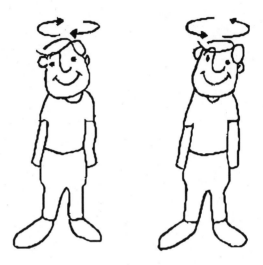

2. With arms down at sides, shrug shoulders up, then relax.

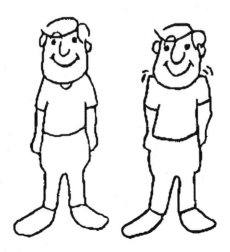

3. Lock hands behind head with elbows pointing forward; take a deep breath in through the nose as you swing elbows back, exhale through the mouth and swing elbows forward.

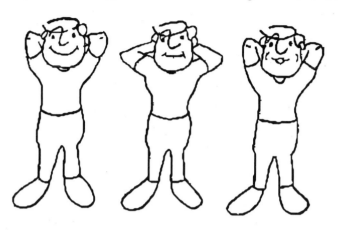

4. With hands on top of shoulders and elbows out to side, make circles with elbows, forward then backward.

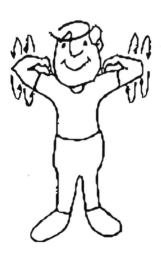

5. With hands on hips, bend trunk side to side.

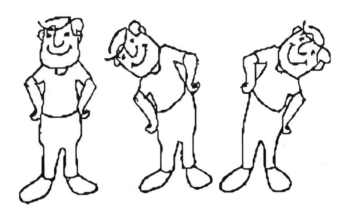

6. With hands in front of chest and arms at shoulder height, twist body from side to side.

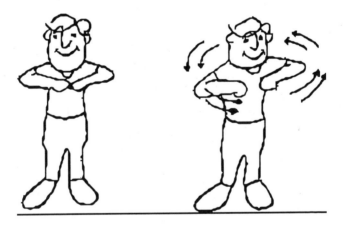

7. With elbows straight, raise arms forward, up over head, and back down.

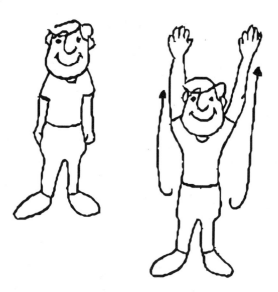

8. With elbows straight, raise arms out to the side, up over head, and back down.

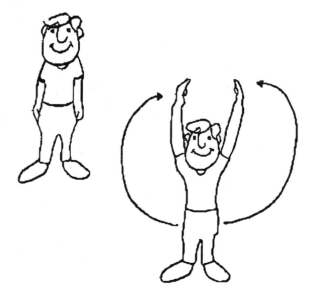

9. Sit comfortably with legs together and straight out in front of you. Point your toes as far as possible and then pull toes back toward your face. Keep knees straight.

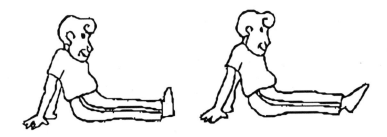

10. Sit with legs together and straight out in front of you. Keeping knees straight, and feet upright, bend forward from the hips and reach toward your feet. Do not dip your head forward--think of bending from the hips without rounding your lower back.

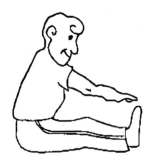

11. Sit with one leg bent and foot against inside of the other leg. Reach toward foot of straight leg, keeping knee down flat and foot upright. Be sure to keep back straight and bend from hip. Reverse leg positions and repeat with opposite leg.

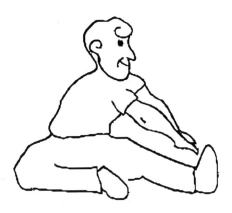

12. Sit with legs spread comfortably apart, knees straight and feet upright. Bend straight forward from the hips, keeping back straight. Do not let knees bend.

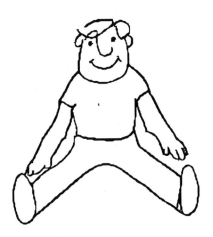

13. Face a wall or something you can lean on for support. Stand with arms in front of you against the support, placing one foot forward and one foot back. Now bend the forward knee and bring it toward the support. The back leg should be straight with the foot flat and pointed straight ahead. (Move back leg forward or back as needed to achieve comfortable stretch on calf). Repeat with opposite leg.

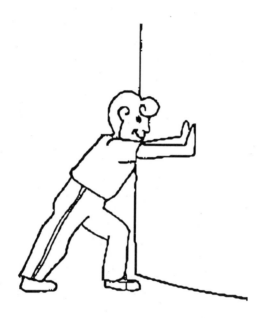

BIBLIOGRAPHY

"Nutritive Value of Foods." U.S. Department of
    Agriculture, Home and Garden Bulletin number 72
"So You Have High Blood Cholesterol." U.S. Department
    of Health and Human Services, National Institutes
    of Health.
"Eating to Lower Your High Blood Cholesterol." U.S.
    Department of Health and Human Services, National
    Institutes of Health.
"Heart Attacks." U.S. Department of Health and Human
    Services, National Institutes of Health.
"Exercise and Weight Control." U.S. Department of
    Health and Human Services.
"Walking for Exercise and Pleasure." U.S. Department
    of Health and Human Services.
"A Consumer's Guide to Food Labels." U.S. Department
    of Health and Human Services, Food and Drug
    Administration.

GLOSSARY

1. <u>ATHEROSCLEROSIS</u> - A type of "hardening of the arteries" in which cholesterol, fat and other blood components build up on the inner lining of arteries. As atherosclerosis progresses, the arteries to the heart may narrow so that oxygen-rich blood and nutrients have difficulty reaching the heart.

2. <u>CALORIE</u> - A unit in which energy is measured. Technically, a calorie is the amount of heat necessary to raise the temperature of a gram of water one degree Centigrade.

3. <u>CARBOHYDRATE</u> - One of three nutrients that supply calories (energy) to the body. Carbohydrate provides 4 calories per gram—the same number of calories as pure protein and less than half the calories of fat. Carbohydrate is essential for normal body function. There are two basic kinds of carbohydrate—simple carbohydrate (or sugars) and complex carbohydrate (starches and fiber). In nature, both the simple sugars and the complex starches come packaged in foods like oranges, apples, corn, wheat, and milk. Refined or processed carbohydrates are found in cookies, cakes, and pies.

3A. <u>COMPLEX CARBOHYDRATE</u> - Starch and fiber. Complex carbohydrate comes from plants. When complex carbohydrate is substituted for saturated fat, the saturated fat reduction helps lower blood cholesterol. Foods high in starch include breads, cereals, pasta, rice, dried beans and peas, corn, and lima beans.

3B. <u>FIBER</u> - A nondigestible type of complex carbohydrate. High-fiber foods are usually low in calories. Foods high in fiber include whole grain breads and cereals, whole fruits, and dried beans. The type of fiber found in foods such as oat and barley bran, some fruits like apples and oranges, and some dried beans may help reduce blood cholesterol.

4. <u>CHOLESTEROL</u> - A soft, waxy substance. It is made in sufficient quantity by the body for normal body function, including the manufacture of hormones, bile acid, and vitamin D. It is present in all parts of the body, including the nervous system, muscle, skin, liver, intestines, heart, etc.

4A. <u>BLOOD CHOLESTEROL</u> - Cholesterol that is manufactured in the liver and absorbed from the food you eat and is carried in the blood for use by all parts of the body. A high level of blood cholesterol leads to atherosclerosis and coronary heart disease. Total cholesterol below 200 mg/dl is considered desirable.

4B. <u>DIETARY CHOLESTEROL</u> - Cholesterol that is in the food you eat. It is present only in foods of animal origin, not in foods of plant origin. Dietary cholesterol, like saturated fat, tends to raise blood cholesterol, which increases the risk for heart disease.

5. <u>CORONARY HEART DISEASE</u> - Heart ailment caused by narrowing of the coronary arteries (arteries that supply oxygen and nutrients directly to the heart muscle). Coronary heart disease is caused by atherosclerosis, which decreases the blood supply to the heart muscle. The inadequate supply of oxygen-rich blood and nutrients may damage the heart muscle and can lead to chest pain, heart attack, and death.

6. <u>FAT</u> - One of the three nutrients that supply calories to the body. Fat provides 9 calories per gram, more than twice the number provided by carbohydrate or protein. In addition to providing calories, fat helps in the absorption of vitamins. Small amounts of fat are necessary for normal body function.

6A. <u>TOTAL FAT</u> - The sum of the saturated, monounsaturated, and polyunsaturated fats present in food. A mixture of all three in varying amounts is found in most foods.

6B. <u>SATURATED FAT</u> - A type of fat found in greatest amounts in foods from animals such as meat, poultry, and whole-milk dairy products like cream, milk, ice cream, and cheese. Other examples of saturated fat include butter, the marbling and fat along the edges of meat, butter and lard. And the saturated fat content is high in some vegetable oils—like coconut, palm kernel, and palm oils. Saturated fat raises blood cholesterol more than anything else in the diet.

6C. <u>UNSATURATED FAT</u> - A type of fat that is usually liquid at refrigerator temperature. Monounsaturated fat and polyunsaturated fat are two kinds of unsaturated fat.

6D. <u>MONOUNSATURATED FAT</u> - (Oleic Acid) A slightly unsaturated fat that is found in greatest amounts in foods from plants, including olive and canola (rapeseed) oil. When substituted for saturated fat, monounsaturated fat helps reduce blood cholesterol.

6E. <u>OMEGA-3 FATTY ACID</u> (FISH OIL) - A type of polyunsaturated fat found in seafood and found in greatest amounts in fatty fish. Seafood is lower in saturated fat than meat.

6F. <u>POLYUNSATURATED FAT</u> - (Linoleic Acid) A highly unsaturated fat that is found in greatest amounts in foods from plants, including safflower, sunflower, corn, and soybean oils. When substituted for saturated fat, polyunsaturated fat helps reduce blood cholesterol.

7. <u>GRAM</u> (g) - A unit of weight. There are about 28 grams in one ounce. Dietary fat, protein, and carbohydrate are measured in grams.

8. <u>HYDROGENATION</u> - A chemical process that changes liquid vegetable oils (unsaturated fat) into more solid saturated fat. This process improves the shelf life of the product—but also increases the saturated fat content. Many commercial food products contain hydrogenated vegetable oil. Selection should be made based on information found on the label.

9. <u>Linoleic Acid</u> - See Fat (Polyunsaturated)
10. <u>LIPOPROTEINS</u> - Protein coated packages that carry fat and cholesterol through the blood. Lipoproteins are classified according to their density.

10A. <u>HIGH DENSITY LIPOPROTEINS</u> (HDL) - Lipoproteins that contain a small amount of cholesterol and carry cholesterol away from body cells and tissues to the liver for excretion from the body. Low levels of HDL are associated with an increased risk of coronary heart disease.

Therefore, the higher the HDL level, the better. Ideal levels are above 35 mg/dl.

10B. <u>LOW DENSITY LIPOPROTEINS</u> (LDL) - Lipoproteins that contain the largest amount of cholesterol in the blood. LDL is responsible for depositing cholesterol in the artery walls. High levels of LDL are associated with an increased risk of coronary heart disease. Ideal levels are below 130 mg/dl.

10C. <u>VERY LOW-DENSITY LIPOPROTEINS</u> (VLDL) - Lipoproteins that are made by the liver and released into the blood. They carry fat to all parts of the body. Ideal levels are below 30 mg/dl.

11. <u>Oleic Acid</u> - See Fat (Monounsaturated)
12. <u>MILLIGRAM</u> (mg) - A unit of weight equal to one-thousandth of a gram. There are about 28,350 mg in 1 ounce. Dietary cholesterol is measured in milligrams.

13. <u>MILLIGRAMS/DECILITER</u> (mg/dl) - A way of expressing concentration: in blood cholesterol measurements, the weight of cholesterol (in milligrams) in a deciliter of blood. A deciliter is about one-tenth of a quart.

14. <u>NUTRIENTS</u> - Components of food that help nourish the body. They provide energy, or help in the maintenance or repair of body tissues, and include carbohydrates, fat, protein, minerals, vitamins and water.

15. <u>PROTEIN</u> - One of the three nutrients that supply calories to the body. Protein provides 4 calories per gram, which is less than half the calories of fat. Protein is an essential nutrient that becomes a component of many parts of the body, including muscle, bone, skin, and blood.

16. <u>TRIGLYCERIDES</u> - Lipids are fat-like substances carried through the bloodstream to the tissues. The bulk of the body's fat tissue is in the form of triglycerides, stored for later use as energy. We get triglycerides primarily from the fat in our diet.

DAILY LOG   DATE _____/_____/_____
ALLOWED--Calories _____ Fat (g) _____ 20 percent
Cholesterol _____ _____ Fat (g) _____ 30 percent

Breakfast	Calories	CHOL.	Fat (g)
_____	_____	_____	_____
_____	_____	_____	_____
_____	_____	_____	_____
_____	_____	_____	_____
_____	_____	_____	_____
_____	_____	_____	_____

Lunch			
_____	_____	_____	_____
_____	_____	_____	_____
_____	_____	_____	_____
_____	_____	_____	_____
_____	_____	_____	_____
_____	_____	_____	_____

Supper			
_____	_____	_____	_____
_____	_____	_____	_____
_____	_____	_____	_____
_____	_____	_____	_____
_____	_____	_____	_____
TOTAL	_____	_____	_____

Percent calories from fat--9 X (_____) total fat grams equals calories from fat (_____) divided by (_____) total calories = _____ percent calories from fat.
Exercise: type _____   time _____
Glasses of water: (8) _____ This amount of water may be too much for some individuals, ask your doctor.

DAILY LOG   DATE _____/_____/_____
ALLOWED--Calories _____ Fat (g) _____ 20 percent
Cholesterol _____ _____ Fat (g) _____ 30 percent

Breakfast	Calories	CHOL.	Fat (g)
_____	_____	_____	_____
_____	_____	_____	_____
_____	_____	_____	_____
_____	_____	_____	_____
_____	_____	_____	_____
Lunch			
_____	_____	_____	_____
_____	_____	_____	_____
_____	_____	_____	_____
_____	_____	_____	_____
_____	_____	_____	_____
Supper			
_____	_____	_____	_____
_____	_____	_____	_____
_____	_____	_____	_____
_____	_____	_____	_____
_____	_____	_____	_____
TOTAL	_____	_____	_____

Percent calories from fat--9 X (_____) total fat grams equals
calories from fat (_____) divided by (_____) total
calories = _____ percent calories from fat.
Exercise: type _____   time _____
Glasses of water: (8) _____ This amount of water may be
too much for some individuals, ask your doctor.

Daily log

DAILY LOG   DATE _____/_____/_____
ALLOWED--Calories _____ Fat (g) _____ 20 percent
Cholesterol _____   _____ Fat (g) _____ 30 percent

Breakfast	Calories	CHOL.	Fat (g)
_____	_____	_____	_____
_____	_____	_____	_____
_____	_____	_____	_____
_____	_____	_____	_____
_____	_____	_____	_____
_____	_____	_____	_____
Lunch			
_____	_____	_____	_____
_____	_____	_____	_____
_____	_____	_____	_____
_____	_____	_____	_____
_____	_____	_____	_____
_____	_____	_____	_____
Supper			
_____	_____	_____	_____
_____	_____	_____	_____
_____	_____	_____	_____
_____	_____	_____	_____
_____	_____	_____	_____
_____	_____	_____	_____
TOTAL	_____	_____	_____

Percent calories from fat--9 X (_____) total fat grams equals calories from fat (_____) divided by (_____) total calories = _____ percent calories from fat.
Exercise: type _____   time _____
Glasses of water: (8) _____ This amount of water may be too much for some individuals, ask your doctor.

244

DAILY LOG   DATE _____/_____/_____
ALLOWED--Calories _____ Fat (g) _____ 20 percent
Cholesterol _____ _____ Fat (g) _____ 30 percent

Breakfast	Calories	CHOL.	Fat (g)
_____	_____	_____	_____
_____	_____	_____	_____
_____	_____	_____	_____
_____	_____	_____	_____
_____	_____	_____	_____
_____	_____	_____	_____
Lunch			
_____	_____	_____	_____
_____	_____	_____	_____
_____	_____	_____	_____
_____	_____	_____	_____
_____	_____	_____	_____
_____	_____	_____	_____
Supper			
_____	_____	_____	_____
_____	_____	_____	_____
_____	_____	_____	_____
_____	_____	_____	_____
_____	_____	_____	_____
_____	_____	_____	_____
TOTAL	_____	_____	_____

Percent calories from fat--9 X (_____) total fat grams equals calories from fat (_____) divided by (_____) total calories = _____ percent calories from fat.
Exercise: type _____   time _____
Glasses of water: (8) _____ This amount of water may be too much for some individuals, ask your doctor.

Index

Index

pulse monitor 127

quality protein 30

rowing machine 130
running 105, 129

safflower oil 72
salt 46
saturated fat 8, 12, 37, 196
Schwinn 131
sedentary 89
sedentary life-style 107
shape 121, 125
shoes 109
simple carbohydrates 25
sodium 46
staple grains 25
starches 25
stationary bicycle 131
step climbing 130
stocky 91
stored fat 93
stretches 111, 172
stretching exercises 99
stroke 8, 106, 161
subcutaneous fat 122
sudden death 46
sugars 25
swimming 130

talk test 118
target heart rate 101
total fat 196
treadmill 131
triglyceride 26
triglycerides 198

unsaturated fat 196

variety 32, 37

very low-density
lipoproteins 197
VLDL 8, 197

walking 105, 111, 129
walking style 109
warm up 115
warmup 172
water 32
whole milk 16

FREE
POSTAGE AND HANDLING

This form required
copies accepted

The
"E-Z-2 READ"
"PERCENT OF CALORIES FROM FAT CHART"
instantly tells you the percent of calories from fat. A must for
everyone trying to limit fat to less than 30% of calories. You
get two sizes, a plastic wallet size for shopping use and a 4x6
magnetic size for quick kitchen reference.

_____ Sets (1 wallet & 1 magnetic)
            $4.00 Per set ....$ _____
_____ Additional wallet size at $1.00 each..............$ _____
_____ Additional magnetic size at $3.00 each.........$ _____
Postage and handling .... **FREE** ....$ --- 0 ---
TOTAL ....$ _____

* *

Enclose your check made out to Readers Choice and mail to:
        READERS CHOICE
        2141 Shaw Ave. Suite 1212
        Clovis, Ca. 93611 - 8916

Allow 4 to 12 weeks for delivery.
PLEASE PRINT - This will be your shipping label.

ORDER YOURS TODAY!
= =

SHIP TO: _____
                _____
                _____
                _____

ORDER TODAY AND **SAVE**
This form required - Copies Accepted

Order direct and save 25 to 30 percent. A great gift for friends
and relatives. Autograph copies available.

* * * **FREE $4.00 Value** * * *

Two "Percent of Calories From Fat" charts for every book
ordered — one wallet size for use in the grocery store and one
4x6 magnetic size for your refrigerator. A four dollar value.—
* * * **FREE!** * * *

"A HEART ATTACK CAN SAVE YOUR LIFE" at $11.96
each (25 % off $15.95 retail price)
[] one book $11.96 plus $3.00 shipping & handling. _____
[] two books $23.92 plus $4.00 S & H ...._____
[] three or more books $11.17 each (**30% OFF**) plus
   only $5.00 shipping & handling ...._____
All books shipped to one address
Allow 4 to 12 weeks for delivery
Two day Priority mail $4.50 per book........................._____
Calif. residents add $0.92 per book sales tax (.077)..._____
[] Autograph copy $1.00 per book. please print
   first name _____ ...._____
TOTAL..._____

Enclose your check made out to Readers Choice and mail to:
       READERS CHOICE
       2141 Shaw Ave. Suite 1212
       Clovis, Ca. 93611 - 8916

PLEASE PRINT - This will be your shipping label.
We will Include **FREE** charts for each book ordered!
ORDER YOURS TODAY!
= =
SHIP TO: _____
             _____
             _____
             _____